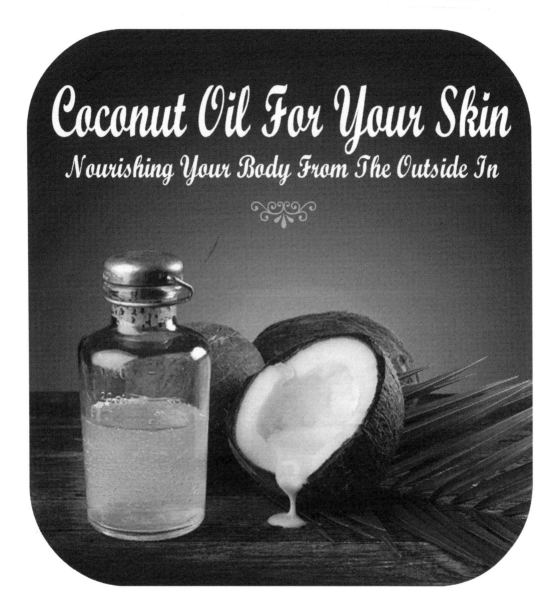

Coconut Oil For Your Skin

Nourishing Your Body From The Outside In

PREFACE

In 2009, I developed a deep love affair with coconut oil! I quickly discovered just how magnificent this oil really is and it became a staple in my home as part of my blossoming real foods lifestyle.

I took my enthusiasm for coconut oil to the public platform and quite accidentally found a voice as an advocate for the many uses of coconut oil through my blog.

I am the author of Hybrid Rasta Mama, a blog which provides my views, experience, insights, and research on any and all things related to conscious parenting, natural/mindful living, holistic health/wellness, real food, and Waldorf education/parenting. My goal is to inspire people around the world to take what I have researched and written, do further research if needed, and apply it to their families and their lives.

This recipe eBook is just the tip of the iceberg. I could write a novel and still not scratch the surface of every recipe and variation. I wanted to provide readers (regardless of your experience making personal care products at home) with an easy-to-use resource that covers some of the basic recipes. I hope you enjoy making them as much as I enjoyed creating them.

To follow my writings, please visit my website, **http://www.hybridrastamama.com**. You can find links to all my social media sites there as well as sign up for my weekly newsletter.

If you are interested in learning more about how coconut oil, coconut milk, coconut water, and coconut meat can improve your health, please frequently check my Coconut Health page: **http://www.hybridrastamama.com/p/coconut-health.html**

Feel free to contact me at jennifer@hybridrastamama.com with any questions, comments, or concerns.

CONTENTS

COCONUT OIL 101

Offering a myriad of health benefits, coconut oil is affordable, readily available, and completely natural. It has hundreds of uses and no harmful or uncomfortable side effects. It is nontoxic to humans and safe to consume and use at any age.

Coconut Oil is:
- Anti-Bacterial
- Anti-Fungal
- Anti-Inflammatory
- Anti-Microbial/Infection Fighting
- Anti-Viral
- An Antioxidant

I encourage you to visit 333 Uses For Coconut Oil to learn more about its benefits and uses.

Since this is a recipe eBook which features Coconut Oil as the star of the show, I want to provide you with *an abbreviated list* which highlights some important ways in which coconut oil can be used for personal hygiene and body care.

Age Spots (also known as liver spots)	Healing for scrapes and cuts
After Shave	Lubricant
Baldness	Makeup Remover
Birth Marks	Massage Oil
Body Scrub	Moisturizer
Bruises	Mole Remover
Bug Bites	Nipple Cream
Burns	Oily Skin Fix
Chapstick	Pre Shampoo Treatment for Hair
Cradle Cap	Pre-Shave
Dandruff	Skin Problems
Deodorant	Stretch Mark Cream
Diaper Salve	Sun Burn Relief
Exfoliator	Sunscreen
Eye cream	Swimmers Ear
Face Wash/ Soap	Tattoo Healing and Moisturizer
Hair Conditioner/ Deep Treatment	Toothpaste
Hair Gel/ Defrizzer	Wrinkle Prevention and Wrinkle Reducer

WHY USE COCONUT OIL FOR PERSONAL CARE PRODUCTS?

There are a lot of choices out there when you are deciding which oil(s) to use in your skincare recipes. However, none compare to the powers of coconut oil. As you saw above, it contains health properties to address a wide variety of external skin-based issues.

Coconut oil is a deeply nourishing oil. The medium chain fatty acids (MC-FAs) contained within coconut oil are quickly and easily absorbed into your skin, where they can be directly utilized for nutrition and energy by the mitochondria (the powerhouse of our cells). This provides all the energy your skin needs to heal, maintain, and flourish.

Using coconut oil in skin care products provides an important layer of protection against skin infections. Other than getting in through natural openings, the only other way fungus and bacteria can enter the body is through weakened spots in the skin. The biggest chemical barrier to infectious organisms is the acid layer on healthy skin. Healthy skin has a pH of about 5, making it slightly acidic. Our sweat (containing uric and lactic acids) and body oils promote this acidic environment, meaning they do us good. Harmless bacteria can tolerate the acid and live on the skin, but troublesome bacteria can't thrive and their numbers are few.

The oil our bodies produce is called sebum. Sebum is secreted by oil glands (sebaceous glands) located at the root of every hair as well as other places. This oil is very important to skin health as it contains MCFAs in the form of medium chain triglycerides that can be released to fight harmful germs. One variety of bacterium that is essential to the healthy environment on our skin converts the medium chain triglycerides (in the sebum or on the skin) into free fatty acids that can kill disease-causing bacteria, viruses, and fungi. This combination of the slightly acid pH and medium chain fatty acids provides a protective chemical layer on the skin that prevents infection from disease-causing organisms. However, when the skin's defenses break down, infections can result.

To better understand coconut oil, here is a peek at the fatty acid profile: 46.45% lauric acid, 20.57% myristic acid, 9.1% palmitic acid, 7.2% oleic acid, 6.6% caprylic acid, 5.07% capric acid, 2.9% stearic acid, and 1.6% linoleic acid. Let's take a look at coconut oil's greatest component, lauric acid.

Lauric acid (an antiseptic fatty acid) present in coconut oil is converted to monolaurin in our body. The effectiveness of monolaurin against microbes which cause skin infections has been tested. It was found that monolaurin has significant sensitivity against a wide range of bacteria which are responsible for superficial skin infections. More importantly, most of the bacteria did not show resistance to the lauric acid in coconut oil, something that cannot be said for many anti-bacterial ingredients.

Coconut oil is also known for its high content of capric acid. Capric acid, much like the lauric acid, is another anti-microbe component. Just like lauric acid, it fights the microbes where they grow and multiply, preventing them from spreading further with hair loss as a result.

The effect of topical application of coconut oil on skin wounds has been studied extensively. It has been found again and again that wounds treated with coconut oil healed much faster, and resulted in an increase in the levels of skin-healing chemicals of the body in the wounded area.

Environmental pollutants, UV light, tobacco smoke, and unhealthy foods cause the development of free radicals in our bodies. These free radicals start destructive chain reactions in our body and damage our cells. After destroying one cell they move on to the next cell. They continue damaging our cells until they are destroyed by antioxidants.

Antioxidants are compounds that neutralize free radicals and stop their destructive chain reactions. Our skin is naturally smooth and elastic because it possesses connective tissues and elastic tissues. During youth these tissues are quite strong making our skin very soft and elastic. As we grow older and become more exposed to our polluted environment, free radicals are formed in our bodies which destroy elastic tissues and cause connective tissues to lose strength. This loosens our skin and results in wrinkles. To combat these devastating free radicals, our bodies need adequate amounts of antioxidants. The Vitamin E, ferulic acid, and p-coumaric acid contained in coconut oil act as strong natural antioxidants.

WHY MAKE YOUR OWN PRODUCTS?

When I started my journey towards living a more natural-minded life, the thought of making my own personal care products seemed really overwhelming. I was worried about sourcing ingredients, cost, time, and quite frankly – goofing up and ending up with a total loss.

I sat down and made a list of pros and cons to making my own products. When I looked at the completed list, I was floored. I literally had four cons and a long list of pros. That sealed the deal. From that day forward there was no turning back; I was sold on making my own personal care products.

I thought that it might be helpful to share the reasons why you should consider making your own personal care products, just in case you are still a little intimidated by the idea.

Let start with the obvious...

Chemicals

Purchase ANY personal care product from the store these days and I can guarantee you that there is something in it that you do not want. When you make your own products, YOU control the ingredients that you are putting onto your skin and ultimately into your body. You can choose ingredients that are environmentally friendly as well as free from dangerous substances.

Let's take a closer look at the dangers of some of the typical chemicals/ preservatives found in today's personal care products:

BHA (butylated hydroxyanisole) and BHT (butylated hydroxytoluene) are closely related synthetic antioxidants used as preservatives in lipsticks and moisturizers, among other cosmetics. BHA is a possible human carcinogen and suspected endocrine disruptor. Both BHA and BHT can induce allergic reactions in the skin. Long-term exposure to high doses of BHT is toxic in mice and rats, causing liver, thyroid, and kidney problems and affecting both lung function and blood coagulation.

DEA (diethanolamine) and DEA compounds are used to make cosmetics creamy or sudsy. DEA also acts as a pH adjuster, counteracting the acidity of other ingredients. DEA is mainly found in moisturizers and sunscreens, while cocamide and lauramide DEA are found in soaps, cleansers, and shampoos. Industrial applications of DEA include its use in oil refineries to "scrub" hydrogen sulphide from process gas emissions. Does that sound like something you want on your skin? DEA and its compounds cause mild to moderate skin and eye irritation. In laboratory experiments, exposure to high doses of these chemicals has been shown to cause liver cancers and precancerous changes in skin and thyroid. Look also for related chemicals MEA and TEA as well.

Parabens are the most widely used preservative in cosmetics. They are also used as fragrance ingredients, but as I mentioned before, consumers won't find that listed on the label as fragrance recipes are considered trade secrets. Parabens easily penetrate the skin. There is evidence that they interfere with hormone function. Parabens can mimic estrogen, the primary female sex hormone. They have been detected in human breast cancer tissues, suggesting a possible association between parabens in cosmetics and cancer. Parabens may also interfere with male reproductive functions. In addition, studies indicate that methylparaben applied on the skin reacts with UVB leading to increased skin aging and DNA damage. Some parabens can trigger allergies and asthma.

Sodium laureth sulfate is used in foaming cosmetics, such as shampoos, cleansers and bubble bath. Depending on manufacturing processes, sodium laureth sulfate may be contaminated with measurable amounts of ethylene oxide, a known human carcinogen, and 1,4-dioxane, a possible human carcinogen. Ethylene oxide can also harm the nervous system and it may interfere with human development. 1,4-dioxane doesn't easily degrade and can remain in the environment long after it is rinsed down the shower drain. In a study of personal care products marketed as "natural" or "organic" (uncertified), U.S. researchers found 1,4-dioxane as a contaminant in 46 of 100 products analyzed. Look also for related chemical sodium lauryl sulfate and other ingredients with the letters "eth" (e.g. Sodium Myreth Sulfate/ Polyethylene Glycol).

Formaldehyde-releasing preservatives: look for the following ingredient names: DMDM hydantoin, diazolidinyl urea, imidazolidinyl urea, methenamine and quarternium-15. These formaldehyde-releasing agents are used as preservatives in a wide range of cosmetics. Other industrial applications of formaldehyde include production of resins used in wood products, vinyl flooring and other plastics, permanent-press fabric, and toilet bowl cleaners. Uh, yuck! These ingredients are a concern because they slowly and continuously release small amounts of formaldehyde, which is a known human carcinogen. Formaldehyde may off-gas from cosmetics containing these ingredients and be inhaled (most of the cancer research on formaldehyde has focused on risks from inhalation). Laboratory studies suggest that formaldehyde in cosmetics can also be absorbed through the skin. DMDM hydantoin and quaternium-15 can irritate skin and eyes and trigger allergies at low doses.

Dibutyl phthalate (pronounced "thal-ate"), or DBP, is used mainly in nail products as a solvent for dyes and as a plasticizer that prevents nail polishes from becoming brittle. Phthalates are also used as fragrance ingredients in many other cosmetics, but consumers won't find these listed on the label. Fragrance recipes are considered trade secrets, so manufacturers are not required to disclose fragrance chemicals in the list of ingredients. DBP is absorbed through the skin. It can enhance the capacity of other chemicals to cause genetic mutations, although it has not been shown to be a mutagen itself. In laboratory experiments, it has been shown to cause developmental defects, changes in the testes and prostate, and reduced sperm count.

The term **"fragrance" or "perfume"** on a cosmetic ingredients list usually represents a complex mixture of dozens of chemicals. Some 3,000 chemicals are used as fragrances. Fragrance is an obvious ingredient in perfumes, colognes, and deodorants, but it's used in nearly every type of personal care product. Even products marketed as "fragrance-free" or "unscented" may in fact contain fragrance along with a masking agent that prevents the brain from perceiving odor. Of the thousands of chemicals used in fragrances, most have not been tested for toxicity (alone or in combination). Many of these unlisted ingredients are irritants and can trigger allergies, migraines, and asthma symptoms. People with multiple chemical sensitivities or environmentally linked illnesses are particularly vulnerable, with fragrances implicated both in development of the condition and triggering symptoms. Synthetic musks used in fragrances are of particular concern from an ecological perspective. Several of musk compounds are persistent in the environment and build up (bioaccumulate) in the fatty tissue of aquatic organisms.

Petrolatum is mineral oil jelly (i.e. petroleum jelly). It is used as a barrier to lock moisture in the skin in a variety of moisturizers and also in hair care products to make your hair shine. As a petroleum product, petrolatum can be contaminated with polycyclic aromatic hydrocarbons (PAHs). Studies suggest that exposure to PAHs is associated with cancer. PAHs in petrolatum can also cause skin irritation and allergies.

PEGs (polyethylene glycols) are petroleum-based compounds that are widely used in cosmetics as thickeners, solvents, softeners, and moisture-carriers. PEGs are commonly used as cosmetic cream bases. They are also used in pharmaceuticals as laxatives. Depending on manufacturing processes, PEGs may be contaminated with measurable amounts of ethylene oxide. (See discussion on ethylene oxide under *Sodium laureth sulfate.*"

PEG compounds themselves show some evidence of genotoxicity, and if used on broken skin can cause irritation and systemic toxicity. Also, PEG functions as a "penetration enhancer," increasing the permeability of the skin to allow greater absorption of the product — including harmful ingredients.

Siloxanes are silicone-based compounds which are used in cosmetics to soften, smooth, and moisten. They make hair products dry more quickly and deodorant creams slide on more easily. They are also used extensively in moisturizers and facial treatments. Siloxanes can also be found in medical implants, water-repellant windshield coatings, building sealants and lubricants. Cyclotetrasiloxane and cylcopentasiloxane (also known as D4 and D5) are toxic, persistent, and have the potential to bioaccumulate in aquatic organisms. They interfere with human hormone function and may impair human fertility. In laboratory experiments, exposure to high doses of D5 has been shown to cause uterine tumours and harm to the reproductive and immune systems. D5 can also influence neurotransmitters in the nervous system. Look for ingredients ending in "-siloxane" or "-methicone."

Triclosan is used mainly in antiperspirants/deodorants, cleansers, and hand sanitizers as a preservative and an anti-bacterial agent. In addition to cosmetics, triclosan is also used as an antibacterial agent in laundry detergent, facial tissues, and antiseptics for wounds, as well as a preservative to resist bacteria, fungus, mildew, and odors in other household products that are sometimes advertised as "anti-bacterial." Triclosan can pass through skin and is suspected of interfering with hormone function (endocrine disruption). The extensive use of triclosan in consumer products may contribute to antibiotic-resistant bacteria.

Coal Tar Dyes: p-phenylenediamine and colors listed as "FD&C Blue/ Red/Yellow No. 1," "Blue 1," or "CI" followed by a five digit number. Coal tar is a mixture of many chemicals, derived from petroleum. P-phenylenediamine is a particular coal tar dye used in many hair dyes. Darker hair dyes tend to contain more phenylenediamine than lighter colors. Coal tar is recognized as a human carcinogen; the main concern with individual coal tar colors (whether produced from coal tar or synthetically) is their potential to cause cancer. As well, these colors may be contaminated with low levels of heavy metals and some are combined with aluminum substrate. Aluminum compounds and many heavy metals are toxic to the brain. Some colors are not approved as food additives, yet they are used in cosmetics that may be ingested, like lipstick.

Allergens

If you are a celiac, you have to be a very savvy label reader not only in the food aisles of your grocery store but also in the toiletry aisles. More often than not, personal care products are made with a ingredients containing gluten. Sadly, it might not even be obvious or it might not even appear in the ingredient list. (There are legal reasons why a company does not have to disclose certain ingredients).

There are all kinds of allergens (chemicals aside) that appear in even the most natural of product brands. Eggs, honey, oats, milk, and certain popular oils are frequently found in store-bought products. Making your own products alleviates the need to read labels and worry over hidden ingredients. You will KNOW what you are putting into your product and that it is not something you will react to.

Overpriced

The companies manufacturing the personal care products sold everywhere are not interested in making them affordable. They want to make money — and lots of it. The natural product lines are not better. In fact, price-point wise, they are worse. They feed off the label of "natural," knowing that consumers will happily plunk out more money since it has fewer or no nasty chemicals and allergens.

I can make my face wash for about $1.00 per bottle and it lasts me 3-4 months. The most natural face wash on the market today runs about $15.99 for a bottle that lasts about 4 months. WHAT? Why would you pay that much when you can make your own? That is insane to me!

Over-Packaged

Not every product is over-packaged but in general, there is either wasted space in the bottle, tube, or jar, or it comes with unnecessary packaging designed to keep the product safe from tampering. Oftentimes you have the main product vessel (let's say a bottle) that has plastic wrap serving as a seal around the screw top. When you remove that, there is the little paper or foam-like seal that you have to remove under the cap so you can use the product. And then you dispose of the bottle when you are done and purchase a new one. Too much waste!

When you make your own products you can reuse the same containers or take advantage of repurposed ones.

Chemicals in the Packaging

BPA anyone? We don't really know how much or which chemicals leach into our products from the packaging; the jury is still out on that one. However, by making your own products at home, you are in charge of what they are stored in and as such, you can make an educated decision on the safest option for you.

Often Made In Factories Owned By Conglomerates With Questionable Ethics

Marketing is a company's greatest asset. Hooking a consumer with clever slogans, targeted messages, and pictures which elicit an emotional response are just a few of the ways they get us comfortable with purchasing their product. Behind the scenes, not every company is truly as ethical as they would appear on paper.

No one REALLY knows what goes on behind closed doors except the employees, owners, and sometimes stakeholders in a company. This is simply not something I am comfortable with. I will never take a company at its word and when possible, I will only support companies I have vetted to the best of my ability. Making my own personal care products allows me to be my own boss, treat my employees fairly (my sweet daughter who always wants to help), and provide outstanding working conditions. I cannot guarantee that this is the case for the employees working for other companies.

Easy and Fun

Mixing up ingredients, experimenting with new butters and oils, and watching a new product come together is actually kind-of a rush! I get a real sense of accomplishment when I successfully create or tweak a recipe.

Once you have gathered all of the ingredients you will need, most recipes are really easy to pull together. It isn't laborious — no drudgery involved. The smells will awaken your senses and pretty soon you will be addicted to the process of making your own personal care products! It really is a lot of fun!

A Great Activity To Do With Your Children

Getting children involved in anything do-it-yourself is both rewarding for them as they develop a passion for creating something with their hands, and it is also very rewarding for your relationship. You will have the chance to make some great memories together as you work side-by-side, creating bath cookies, shampoos, salves, and other products. Do you want your children to remember a shopping trip to the local big-box store or the time they spent with you, creating something that will nourish the body from the outside in?

INGREDIENTS

CARRIER OILS AND BUTTERS

In natural skin care, carrier oils are typically referred to as vegetable oils, fixed oils, or base oils. However, not all fixed oils/base oils are vegetable oils. Emu oil (from the emu bird) and fish (marine) oils are also classified as fixed/base oils, but these animal-based oils are generally not used for personal care products.

Vegetable butters are similar to vegetable carrier oils but they are solid at room temperature. Vegetable butters are processed by a wide variety of methods, so it's especially important to check the method of extraction when shopping for butters. Strive to use butters that are cold pressed. Cocoa butter and shea butter are the most widely used.

Here are the carrier oils and butters you will find in the recipes presented here:

Avocado Oil – The oil from avocados is very rich and one of the most moisturizing. It contains Vitamins A, D, and E, all of which are beneficial. This oil is a great choice for those with older or extremely dry, itchy skin. This is a medium weight oil with a light green hue that absorbs well.

Fatty Acid Profile: 75-80% oleic acid 7-10%, up to 4% stearic acid, and up to 10% palmitic acid.

Shelf Life: 12 months.

Almond Oil (Sweet Almond Oil) – This oil is high in protein and offers moisturizing, softening, and regenerating properties. It can also act as an anti-inflammatory ingredient, helping to restore and repair our skin barrier. This is a wonderful oil for those with dry, itchy skin. It is light, odorless, and absorbs well.

Fatty Acid Profile: 60-78% oleic acid, 10-30% linoleic acid, 3-9% palmitic acid, 2% palmitoleic acid, 3% stearic acid, and 2% linolenic acid.

Shelf Life: 12 months.

Apricot Kernel Oil – This oil is a rich and soothing emollient which offers softening, regenerating, and moisturizing properties, as well as some anti-inflammatory properties thanks to its oleic acid content. The linoleic acid contained in apricot kernel oil offers support to skin barrier repair and can help with dry, itchy skin. This is a light oil with little to no scent that is absorbed quickly and easily by the skin.

Fatty Acid Profile: 58-74% oleic acid, 20-34% linoleic acid, 4-7% palmitic acid, and 1% stearic acid.

Shelf Life: 12 months.

Borage Oil – This is a powerhouse oil. The fatty acid profile gives it some of the most extensive healing powers. This oil can help with moisture retention, flexibility of the skin, cell regeneration, and skin repair. It will help restore barrier function of our skin, and acts as an anti-inflammatory that can soothe dry skin and itchiness. In addition, it has some powerful antioxidants in the form of ferulic acid, which will prevent skin aging, reduce age spots, and help to repair light- and radiation-induced skin damage. It penetrates the skin easily but the tannins found in borage oil make it a more astringent oil so it will feel a bit drier on your skin.

Fatty Acid Profile: 36% linoleic acid, 23% gamma linolenic acid , 17% oleic acid, 11% stearic acid, 4% palmitic acid, 4% gadoleic acid, 2% erucic acid, and 2% nervonic acid.

Shelf Life: 6 months.

Castor Oil – This oil offers some anti-inflammatory and itch reducing properties. The ricinoleic acid is considered an analgesic and is antibacterial, and there are some indications it might act as an antifungal. It has skin softening benefits. This is a very thick oil, pale in color, with very little scent. It penetrates the skin easily but can be greasy or sticky which is why it is used in such low amounts.

Fatty Acid Profile: 85-90% ricinoleic acid, 4% linoleic acid, and 2-6% oleic acid.

Shelf Life: 12 months.

Cocoa Butter – This butter is water repellent and very protective. It acts as a barrier ingredient that provides an occlusive layer on our skin which reduces the amount of water lost from our skin and protects it from the elements. It offers a lot of skin softening benefits, cell regenerating benefits, as well as anti-inflammatory effects. It even has some natural sun-blocking qualities. Cocoa butter will make anything you use it in a little thicker.

Fatty Acid Profile: 34-36% oleic acid, 31-35% stearic acid, 25-30% palmitic acid, and 3% linoleic acid.

Shelf Life: 2-5 years.

Grape Seed Oil – This oil is one of the least greasy feeling oils. It is ideal for those with oily skin and is also used in protective creams such as sunscreens and sunblocks. Grape Seed Oil is anti-microbial, has high antioxidant properties and is known to help with barrier repair, reduction of inflammation, and reduction of itching.

Fatty Acid Profile: 72% linoleic acid, 16% oleic acid, 7% palmitic, and 4% stearic acid.

Shelf Life: 3-6 months.

Hazelnut Oil – This oil is a great emollient. Due to the high Vitamin E content, hazelnut oil is absorbed quickly by the skin, offering softening and moisturizing benefits. It can offer some mild UV protection and it has cell regenerative properties. It also contains quite a few minerals like potassium, calcium, and magnesium. Hazelnut oil is a "dry oil," meaning you cannot feel it on your skin.

Fatty Acid Profile: 66-85% oleic acid, up to 25% linoleic acid, 4-9% palmitic acid, and 1-4% stearic acid.

Shelf Life: 12 months.

Hemp Seed Oil – This oil reduces itchiness, redness, and inflammation. The carotenoids it contains may offer anti-inflammatory benefits to a product. It is cell regenerating, helpful in restoring barrier properties, retains moisture, and offers softening properties. This is another dry oil that is easily absorbed and barely noticeable on the skin.

Fatty Acid Profile: 57% linoleic acid, 19-25% linolenic acid , 12% oleic acid, 6% palmitic acid, up to 5% gamma linolenic acid, and 2% stearic acid.

Shelf Life: 3-6 months, but certain brands have a shelf life of up to 12 months.

Jojoba Oil – This oil is different from most vegetable oils in that it is not made up of fat but of liquid wax. It is ideal for cosmetic use because of its molecular stability and its natural moisturizing and healing characteristics. It promotes improved moisture retention, flexibility of the skin, and skin repair. Jojoba oil sinks quickly into the skin as it penetrates through hair follicles, but it does not block the follicles in the process. Jojoba actually mixes with the sebum on our bodies to create a thin non-occlusive layer of jojoba oil and sebum.

Fatty Acid Profile: 57% gadoleic acid, 20% erucic acid, 14% oleic acid, 7% stearic acid, 2% palmitic acid.

Shelf Life: 2 years.

Mango Butter – This butter offers great moisturizing and softening of your skin by being well absorbed by the skin. It contains Vitamins A, B, and C, making it anti-inflammatory, anti-fungal, anti-bacterial, and a powerful antioxidant.

Fatty Acid Profile: 46% oleic acid, 42% stearic acid, 6% palmitic acid, and 3% linoleic acid.

Shelf Life: 2-3 years.

Neem Oil – This oil is actually steam distilled from the leaves and seeds of a tree found in Asia, India, Indonesia, and tropical areas of Australia. It is dark brown in color and has a strong scent. The neem tree is known as a living pharmacy because of its variety of medicinal benefits. It is now being used by practitioners worldwide for various treatments including skin conditions. Neem oil is rich in essential fatty acids that nourish and balance problem skin. The natural oils and glycerides quickly and easily penetrate outer layers of skin to soothe even chronically dry, itchy, or flaking areas.

Neem oil contains both potent anti-oxidants and essential fatty acids, making it very effective for smoothing wrinkles and fine lines while helping to prevent the signs of aging when used regularly. It has been traditionally used to even out skin tone irregularities, helping to balance and restore proper skin pigmentation for issues such as vitiligo or age spots.

Fatty Acid Profile: 52% oleic acid, 21% stearic acid, 12% palmitic acid, 2% lineolaic acid.

Shelf Life: 2 years.

Olive Oil – This oil is moisturizing, regenerating, softening, offers anti-inflammatory properties, and is well absorbed by the skin. It also promotes vitamin D synthesis in our bodies. Olive oil helps to repair damaged cells and increase cell regeneration.

Fatty Acid Profile: 55-83% oleic acid, 10.5% palmitic acid, 4-21% linoleic acid, 2.6% stearic acid, and 1% linolenic acid.

Shelf Life: 12 months.

Shea Butter – This butter has high levels of vitamins A & E, and provides nourishment to both skin and hair by revitalizing and softening without leaving a greasy residue. It reduces irritation and redness, protects skin, regenerates cells, heals wounds, moisturizes, prevents premature aging, and acts as a sunscreen.

Fatty Acid Profile: 40-55% oleic acid, 35-45% stearic acid, 3-7% palmitic acid, and 3-8% linoleic acid.

Shelf Life: 2 years.

Sunflower Oil – This is a light oil that is absorbed easily. It is known for softening of the skin, alleviation of dry skin, and it also has anti-inflammatory benefits!

Fatty Acid Profile: 61-73% linoleic acid, 16-36% oleic acid, 5-7% palmitic acid, and 3-6% stearic acid.

Shelf Life: 3-6 months.

Essential Oils

Essential oils are pure aromatic plant essences. They are distilled from flowers, fruit, leaves, resins, roots, seeds, and wood. They are used for their healing properties all over the world.

Although essential oils have many benefits, only some of the essential oils available are suitable for children. Others are not suitable for children and some are even dangerous to children. Please research essential oil safety before using any of these products on children.

Whenever you are working with essential oils, please use caution. Essential oils should never be applied undiluted directly on the skin. They are also flammable. Less is more!

Some oils may cause sensitivity or an allergic reaction, so it is advisable to test for sensitivity: mix one drop of the essential oil with one tablespoon of a carrier oil and apply it to the inside of your wrist. Wait 24 hours. If no reaction occurs then the chances of a skin sensitivity are slim.

Below is a chart listing the most commonly used essential oils along with both the physical and mental/emotional ailments aided. This is intended to serve as a guide when making a selection of which essential oil to include in your recipes.

Essential Oil	Physical	Mental
Angelica root	Dull skin, gout, psoriasis, toxin build-up, water retention	Exhaustion, nervousness, and stress
Anise	Bronchitis, colds, coughs, flatulence, flu, muscle aches, rheumatism	Depression
Basil	Bronchitis, colds, coughs, exhaustion, flatulence, flu, gout, insect bites, insect repellent, muscle aches, rheumatism and sinusitis	Fatigue, exhaustion, burnout, memory and concentration
Bay	Dandruff, hair care, neuralgia, oily skin, poor circulation, sprains and strains	Emotional exhaustion and fatigue
Bergamot	Acne, abscesses, anxiety, boils, cold sores, cystitis, halitosis, itching, loss of appetite, oily skin, psoriasis	Anger, anxiety, confidence, depression, stress, fatigue, fear, peace, happiness, insecurity and loneliness
Cardamom	Appetite loss of, colic, halitosis	Fatigue, stress, shame, guilt
Carrot Seed	Eczema, gout, mature skin, toxin build-up, water retention	Anxiety, confusion, exhaustion, mood swings and stress
Cedarwood	Acne, arthritis, bronchitis, coughs, cystitis, dandruff, dermatitis, insect repellent, stress	Anxiety, fear, and insecurity
Cedarwood Atlas	Acne, arthritis, bronchitis, coughing, cystitis, dandruff and dermatitis	Anxiety, fear, insecurity, and stress
German Chamomile	Abscesses, allergies, arthritis, boils, colic, cuts, cystitis, dermatitis, dysmenorrhea, earache, flatulence, hair care, headache, inflamed skin, insect bites, insomnia, nausea, neuralgia, PMS, rheumatism, sores, sprains, strains, wounds	Anger, anxiety, depression, fear, irritability, loneliness, and stress
Roman Chamomile	Abscesses, allergies, arthritis, boils, colic, cuts, cystitis, dermatitis, dysmenorrhea, earache, flatulence, hair care, headache, inflamed skin, insect bites, nausea, neuralgia, PMS, rheumatism, sores, sprains, strains, wounds	Anger, anxiety, depression, fear, irritability, loneliness, insomnia, stress

Essential Oil	Physical	Mental
Cinnamon	Constipation, exhaustion, flatulence, lice, low blood pressure, rheumatism, scabies	Concentration, emotional and mental fatigue
Citronella	Excessive perspiration, fatigue, headache, insect repellent, oily skin	Mind fog, tension
Clary Sage	Amenorrhea, asthma, coughing, gas, labor pains, sore throat	Anxiety, fatigue, exhaustion, fear, loneliness and stress
Clove	Arthritis, asthma, bronchitis, immune system, rheumatism, sprains, toothache	Memory and concentration, fatigue, depression
Coriander	Aches, arthritis, colic, gout, indigestion, nausea, rheumatism	Fatigue, irritation
Cypress	Excessive perspiration, hemorrhoids, oily skin, rheumatism, varicose veins.	Confidence, grief, memory and concentration
Eucalyptus	Arthritis, bronchitis, catarrh, cold sores, colds, coughing, fever, flu, poor circulation, sinusitis	Concentration and memory
Fennel	Bruises, cellulite, flatulence, bleeding gums, halitosis, mouth, nausea, obesity, toxin build-up, water retention	Fatigue, emotional imbalance
Frankincense	Anxiety, asthma, bronchitis, extreme coughing, scars and stretch marks	Anxiety, depression, fatigue exhaustion and burnout, fear, grief, happiness and peace, insecurity, loneliness, panic and panic attacks, and stress
Geranium	Acne, cellulite, dull skin, lice, menopause, oily skin.	Anxiety, depression, happiness, mood imbalance and stress
Ginger	Aching muscles, arthritis, nausea, poor circulation	Fatigue, exhaustion and burnout
Grapefruit	Cellulite, dull skin, toxin build-up, water retention	Confidence, fear, depression, happiness and peace, stress
Helichrysum	Abscesses, acne, boils, burns, cuts, dermatitis, eczema, irritated skin, wounds	Grief, loneliness, panic and panic attacks, shock

Essential Oil	Physical	Mental
Hyssop	Bruises, coughing, sore throat, respiratory system	Concentration, nervousness
Jasmine	Dry skin, labor pains, sensitive skin	Stress, depression, fear
Lavender	Acne, allergies, anxiety, asthma, athlete's foot, bruises, burns, chicken pox, colic, cuts, dermatitis, earache, flatulence, headache, hypertension, insect bites, insect repellent, itching, labor pains, migraine, oily skin, rheumatism, scabies, scars, sores, sprains/strains, stress, stretch marks, vertigo	Anxiety, depression, irritability, panic attacks, stress
Lemon	Athlete's foot, colds, corns, dull skin, flu, oily skin, spots, varicose veins, warts	Fear happiness and peace, memory and concentration
Lemon Grass	Acne, athlete's foot, digestion, excessive perspiration, flatulence, insect repellent, muscle aches, oily skin, scabies, stress	Fatigue and mental confusion
Marjoram	Aching muscles, arthritis, cramps, migraine, neuralgia, rheumatism, spasm, sprains	Mood swings, PMS symptoms, stress
Melissa	Flu, indigestion, herpes, nausea, shingles and cold sores	Agitation, anxiety, dementia, nervous tension
Myrrh	Amenorrhea, athlete's foot, bronchitis, chapped skin, bleeding gums, halitosis, itching, ringworm	Emotional imbalance, creativity
Myrtle	Acne, asthma, coughs, hemorrhoids, irritated skin	Addiction and self-destructive behavior, depression
Neroli	Mature skin, oily skin, scars, stretch marks	Anxiety, depression, anger, irritability, panic attacks, stress
Nutmeg	Arthritis, constipation, muscle aches, nausea, neuralgia, poor circulation, rheumatism, slow digestion	Mental fatigue
Bitter Orange	Colds, constipation, dull skin, flatulence, flu, bleeding gums, mouth, slow digestion	Anger, confidence, depression, fear, happiness, peace, stress

Essential Oil	Physical	Mental
Oregano	Coughs, digestion, respiration	Insecurity
Parsley	Congestion, digestion, diuretic, immune system, kidney infections and stones	Frigidity
Patchouli	Acne, cellulite, chapped skin, dandruff, dermatitis, eczema, mature skin, oily skin	Fatigue, frigidity, exhaustion, stress
Peppermint	Asthma, colic, exhaustion, fever, flatulence, headache, nausea, scabies, sinusitis, vertigo	Fatigue, exhaustion and burnout, memory and concentration
Rose	Eczema and mature skin	Anger, anxiety, frigidity, depression grief, menopause, happiness and peace, loneliness, panic and panic attacks, stress
Rosemary	Aching muscles, arthritis, dandruff, dull skin, exhaustion, gout, hair care, muscle cramping, neuralgia, poor circulation, rheumatism	Fatigue, exhaustion and burnout, confidence, memory and concentration
Sandalwood	Bronchitis, chapped and dry skin, laryngitis, oily skin, strep throat, urinary tract problems	Anxiety, depression, exhaustion and burnout, fear, grief, irritability, stress
Spearmint	Asthma, exhaustion, flatulence, headache, nausea, scabies	Depression and mental fatigue
Thyme	Arthritis, bronchitis, candida, cuts, dermatitis, gastritis, laryngitis	Concentration and memory
Violet Leaf	Bronchitis, insomnia, liver congestion, sluggish circulation, problem skin	Fear, nostalgia, obsession, shyness
Yarrow	Acne, arthritis, inflammation, hair care, hypertension, insomnia	Insomnia, stress and tension
Ylang Ylang	Hypertension, menopause and PMS symptoms, palpitations	Anger, depression, frigidity, mood swings, PMS, stress

OTHER INGREDIENTS

Aloe Vera - Several properties of the aloe vera plant make it an excellent remedy for speeding up the healing process for treating scars, burns, and cuts. It is well known for its anti-inflammatory properties and it has both antibacterial and antifungal effects. It is a cellular regenerator and a strong antioxidant.

Beeswax - Forms a light barrier on your skin, helping to seal in moisture without clogging pores. Beeswax offers anti-inflammatory, antibacterial, and antiviral benefits. It also contains vitamin A, which may be beneficial in softening and hydrating dry skin and in cell reconstruction. Beeswax is typically used as a thickening agent.

Coconut Milk - One of the best liquid ingredients you can put on your skin! Some of its known benefits are:

- Helps to form a chemical barrier on the skin to ward of infection.
- Reduces symptoms associated the psoriasis, eczema, and dermatitis.
- Supports the natural chemical balance of the skin.
- Softens skin and helps relieve dryness and flaking.
- Prevents wrinkles, sagging skin, and age spots.
- Promotes healthy looking hair and complexion.
- Provides protection from damaging effects of ultraviolet radiation from the sun.
- Helps control dandruff.

Flaxseed Oil - A rich source of healing compounds. The essential fatty acids in flaxseed oil are largely responsible for its skin-healing powers. Red, itchy patches of eczema, psoriasis, and rosacea often respond to the EFAs' anti-inflammatory actions and overall skin-soothing properties. Sunburned skin may heal faster when treated with the oil as well. In cases of acne, the EFAs encourage thinning of the oily sebum that clogs pores.

The abundant omega-3 fatty acids in flaxseed oil have been shown to contribute to healthy hair. Hair problems exacerbated by psoriasis or eczema of the scalp may respond to the skin-revitalizing and anti-inflammatory actions of flaxseed oil as well. Similarly, the oil's EFAs work to nourish dry or brittle nails, stopping them from cracking or splitting.

Green Tea - Numerous health benefits; an excellent additive to any skin care product. It fights free radicals which increases the antioxidant capacity of tissues and blood. It has been proven that products based on the extract of this type of tea reverse the aging process at the cellular level. A number of studies have indicated that green tea extract neutralizes the harmful effects of UV on human skin.

Green tea is rich in polyphenols which fight free radicals (the leading causes of cellular mutations leading to skin cancer). Because of its components, it is a potent anti-inflammatory agent. People who suffer from skin diseases like psoriasis, dandruff, rosacea, or skin sensitivity can benefit from its calming effect. In addition to the beneficial properties already mentioned above, the catechins in green tea are anti-bacterial and they also regulate hormonal activity. Therefore, it is very beneficial for acne prone skin.

Honey - Often used as a preservative in natural skincare products. It has been found to be a wound healer, antiseptic, a great moisturizer, and it is also soothing and softening to skin. The antibacterial properties in honey help in fighting acne and pimples. It soaks up impurities from the pores of the skin, leaving your skin clear and clean. Honey is also antiseptic. When honey is diluted with water, it produces hydrogen peroxide making it useful in treating cuts, wounds, and abrasions. Honey also protects your skin while in the sun and assists the skin to rejuvenate and stay young.

Lanolin - Its molecular structure most closely resembles that of human skin. It creates a breathable barrier, so it protects and absorbs at the same time. And once it penetrates into the skin, it holds up to 400 times its weight in water, so it's a fantastic moisture reservoir for skin.

Liquid Glycerin - Glycerin is called glycerol or glycerine as well and is present in all natural lipids (fats), whether animal or vegetable. Glycerin plays a very important role in our skin structure as it is found in large quantities between the three layers of our skin. It enters the blood stream whenever the body requires energy and uses up the stored fats. It also contributes towards cell metabolism. It absorbs water or moisture from the air due to its hygroscopic nature which is why it is known for making skin more supple. It has wound healing properties and is known for aiding in the healing of a large number of skin conditions.

Vitamin E - A thick, rich oil that is used as a natural preservative. Its antioxidant properties help keep oils from going rancid. It's a great wound healer, it fights skin damage, heals scar tissue and stretch marks, moisturizes, and is often used to treat wrinkles and fine lines. Treats dermatitis, wounds, burns, scrapes, and rashes.

VEGAN ALTERNATIVES

In any recipes which call for beeswax, you are welcome to use any of the following alternatives:

- **Candelilla wax** is a plant based wax made by boiling the leaves and stems of the candelilla shrub. It produces something almost identical in texture to beeswax with a very low concentration of sulphuric acid. If you choose to use candelilla wax, you will *only need HALF as much* as the beeswax called for in the recipe. It also hardens much faster than beeswax.

- **Carnauba wax** is another vegan beeswax alternative. It comes from palm trees, though, so make sure your source it carefully as there are many ethical concerns surrounding how palm oil is harvested. If you choose to use carnauba wax, you will *only need HALF as much* as the beeswax called for in the recipe. It also hardens much faster than beeswax.

- **Soy wax** is a great alternative. However, it is important that you only use organic soy wax. If it is not organic it is likely genetically modified. Soy wax can substituted for beeswax at a 1:1 ratio.

- **Bayberry wax** is a plant based wax typically processed by boiling the berries of the wax myrtle shrub then skimming the filmy substance from the surface. It has a strong aroma. If you don't mind the scent, then it makes a great alternative to beeswax and can be substituted for it at a 1:1 ratio.

INGREDIENT NOTES

TYPES OF COCONUT OIL

There are a lot of brands of coconut oil on the market today. While most brands will offer health benefits, not all coconut oil is created equal. Below are the types of coconut oil on the market today. Make sure you read the label carefully. If the label isn't clear, call the company. A reputable company will answer any questions you have. You can also visit Appendix B: Where to Purchase Quality Ingredients for coconut oil I have vetted and trust completely.

Unrefined (AKA virgin or extra-virgin) – this coconut oil comes from fresh coconuts and has not been changed with heat processes. It is the purest, most natural, least processed (chemically-changed) form. You can use it for anything but it will impart a coconut odor (mild and pleasant in my book)! Unrefined coconut oil retains the most beneficial health properties and is superior to refined oil.

Refined (AKA RBD) – manufacturers *typically* do not use fresh coconut and instead use the copra (dry coconut flakes). These flakes are then refined, bleached, and deodorized leaving behind an oil that is colorless, tasteless and odorless. Not all refined coconut oils are alike! Most are refined using a chemical distillation process dependent on lye or other harsh solvents. Know your supplier. While refined coconut oil is almost as beneficial as its unrefined/virgin counterpart, it does lose some (but not all) of its health properties during the refining process.

Fractionated – this coconut oil is one in which manufacturers remove all of the long-chain fatty acids (and even the medium-chain lauric acid) to retain only its fraction of caprylic and capric acid. They do this to lower its melting point so people can use the oil in liquid form. Fractionated is used most often as a superfatting oil in soaps; in skin-care lotions, cream and similar products as an emollient; in massage oil blends (famous for not staining the sheets); as a carrier oil for essential oils, vitamins and actives; and in medicines.

Cold-Pressed, Expeller-Pressed, and Centrifuged – these are simply names of the various methods of extracting the oil from the dry or fresh coconut and can be found in both refined and unrefined varieties.

Any of the above mentioned coconut oils are just fine to use in any of these recipes! However, I always prefer to use unrefined to ensure that I am getting ALL of the beneficial health properties.

Some General Notes

The carrier oils that you purchase should be natural and unadulterated. Virgin, extra virgin, unrefined, cold pressed, expeller pressed, raw, and organic are labels to look for.

As mentioned above, coconut oil can cause some, but not all, of your products to set like butter or become harder than you would like. Five to ten minutes before using your product, simply place the product container in a bowl of warm water. This will allow the coconut oil to soften slightly, making a more creamy consistency.

When using essential oils it is imperative that you find a reputable supplier of therapeutic-grade essential oils, using organic or wildcrafted varieties when possible. Synthetic copies of oils commonly used in perfumery are not appropriate, and may even be harmful to you or your child's health.

Essential oils will absorb into wood and some plastics. When mixing ingredients, it is best to do so in a glass or steel bowl with a metal spoon.

It is important to note that recipes using cocoa butter or shea butter can cause a slightly gritty texture to occur. This is perfectly normal and safe. The "grit" will actually smooth out as you apply the cream or lotion. You can also lessen the grittiness by cooking the butter over the lowest heat setting for 15 minutes.

Remember – these recipes are free of additives, preservatives, and chemicals, which means that they will not *look* like the products you purchase from the store. However, they will feel so much better and your skin will thank you for only using products from nature.

Be sure to use caution in the bathtub or shower. Any products that contain oil might make the surface areas a bit slippery!

Never microwave coconut oil to melt it! Microwaves destroy all of the beneficial properties. Instead, place the desired amount of coconut oil in a mason jar, glass bowl, or glass measuring cup. Place the glass jar/bowl/cup in a shallow pan of just boiled water, and it will melt fairly quickly.

Storage for Ingredients

Carrier oils can become rancid over time. The level of natural fatty acids, tocopherols, method of extraction and other characteristics of an oil all can affect how quickly an oil becomes rancid. If you come across a carrier oil that has a strong, bitter aroma, the carrier oil may have gone rancid. If you can, compare the aroma of the oil that you suspect is rancid with the same oil that you know is fresh.

Here are a few tips to reduce the chance of rancidity in your carrier oils:

1. If you plan on using all of the oil quickly and long before its lifespan would be reached, then there are no special storage considerations. If you will be keeping them longer, or just have a very fragile carrier oil, then they should be transferred to a dark glass or plastic bottle with a tight fitting top and stored in a dark (always out of direct sunlight) and cool area.

2. Another tip is to put the oil into a smaller container as the level of oil goes down in the bottle, to reduce the amount of air at the top. This will also reduce the chances of rancidity.

3. Most carrier oils can be stored in the refrigerator, especially those with a high gamma linoleic acid content (fat content). Refrigeration is especially helpful for fragile oils such as borage and carrot. The more stable carrier oils (like castor, palm kernel, shea butter, sunflower, olive, almond, and jojoba) do well in a cupboard. *Please note that some oils, like coconut, avocado, and jojoba, will become cloudy and solidify when cold but this does not harm the oils or mean they are rancid.*

Although essential oils do not become rancid, they can oxidize, deteriorate, and lose their beneficial therapeutic properties over time. Oils such as the citrus oils will oxidize and begin to lose their aroma and therapeutic properties in as little as six months. Not all essential oils diminish in quality as time passes. Essential oils such as patchouli and sandalwood mature with age. All essential oils, however, will benefit from proper storage and handling. Here are some storage tips for essential oils:

1. To avoid deterioration and to protect the aromatic and therapeutic properties of your essential oils, store them in amber or cobalt blue bottles. Dark glass such as amber or cobalt helps to keep out deteriorating sunlight. Be leery of purchasing any oils sold in clear glass bottles. Clear glass bottles are not harmful to essential oils, but clear glass does not protect the oils from damaging sunlight.

2. Avoid purchasing pure essential oils sold in plastic bottles as the essential oil will eat at the plastic, and the essential oil will become ruined in a short period of time. Some vendors sell oils in lined aluminum bottles. It has been said that aluminum bottles are acceptable if the interior of the bottles are lined.

3. Essential oils should also be stored in a cool, dark place.

Avoid purchasing essential oils that are stored in bottles that have a rubber dropper incorporated into its screw-top cap. Droppers with rubber bulbs should not be kept with the essential oil bottle as the highly concentrated oil can turn the rubber bulb into gum and ruin the essential oil.

Many essential oils are sold in bottles that contain an "orifice reducer." An orifice reducer is a small, usually clear insert inside the bottle opening that acts as a dropper. Unlike rubber droppers, orifice reducers will not harm essential oils. You simply tip the bottle to dispense the oil drop by drop.

STORAGE FOR FINISHED PRODUCTS

Unless otherwise noted, products do not need refrigeration and can be safely stored in glass jars or another suitable sealed container for up to six months. Most will last longer but use your own discretion.

Ideally, all products should be stored in a cool, dry location and away from direct sunlight.

There are a lot of options for storage vessels. You can use repurposed glass jars (Mason jars and baby food jars are perfect!). A quick trip to a thrift store or garage sale might yield you some really cool looking jars. (Just be conscious that some older jars might contain lead). Old cosmetics bottles can work too, but I am personally leery of reusing anything plastic. You can also order special containers like the ones found at Mountain Rose Herbs. Really, do what works best for your budget and space available! There is no right or wrong vessel to store your products in, just good, better, best.

THE RECIPES

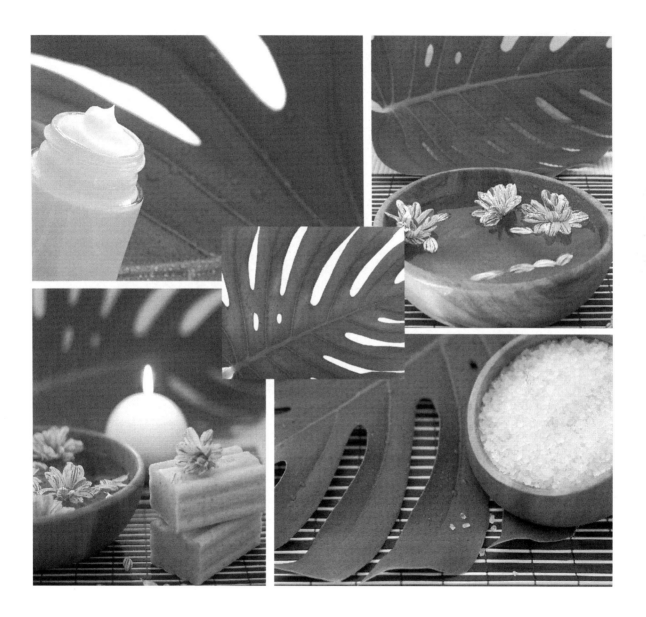

MELTING MADE EASY

Whenever a recipe calls for you to melt any of the oils, butters, or wax, you can use a few different methods. Throughout the recipe section of this book, I will refer to the "mason jar" method (outlined below) but you can substitute any of the other methods based on what you have on hand. I have also included the classic double boiler method, small pot on low heat method, and glass bowl in a pan method.

MASON JAR METHOD

This is by far the simplest method for melting your oils and butters. You can reuse the same jar again and again and you don't have to worry if the jar stays a bit greasy after cleaning. You will be using it to melt more oils and butters so it is ok if a little is left over in the jar.

- Take a glass mason jar (one quart is typically the perfect size) and place it in a small pot.
- Pour enough water around the mason jar so that it reaches about halfway up the sides of the jar. DO NOT GET WATER IN THE JAR!
- Add the ingredients you need to melt to the mason jar, turn the heat on medium-low, and watch the magic happen!
- Be careful not to get the contents of the mason jar wet. (This is why you pour the water around the jar before adding the ingredients.) I like to play it safe by covering the top of the jar with a small plate or even the lid put on loosely.

DOUBLE BOILER METHOD

This is a very easy method, requiring only your double boiler. (I recommend stainless steel). You can even designate the "top" pot for use as your *oil and butter melting pot* which would allow for less pot scrubbing time during clean up. Again, it is alright if your pot has a leftover layer of grease on it from the melted oils and butters.

- Fill the bottom pot with water and place the top pot inside.
- Bring the water to a gentle, rolling boil and add your oils and butters to the top pot.

SMALL POT METHOD

This is another simple method, requiring only one small to medium pot. (Again, I recommend stainless steel). The downside to this method is that you can easily burn the ingredients if you are not careful. The upside is that you can designate this pot for use as your *oil and butter melting pot* which would cut down on clean up time. Again, it is ok if your pot has a leftover layer of grease on it from the melted oils and butters.

- Turn your stove top on low.

- Add your oils and butters as called for in the recipe.

- Stir these constantly as they melt, making sure that the oils and butters never get to the stage of bubbling. You want them melted, not boiling.

GLASS BOWL METHOD

This is a similar method for melting your oils and butters as the mason jar method. You can reuse the same glass bowl again and again and you don't have to worry if the bowl stays a bit greasy after cleaning. Since you will be using it to melt more oils and butters later, it doesn't matter if a little is left over in the bowl. The only downside to this is finding a large enough pot to fit the bowl and making sure that the bowl is covered as the boiling water underneath will easily splash in.

- Take a glass bowl and place it in a medium pot.

- Pour enough water around the bowl so that it reaches about half-way up the sides. DO NOT GET WATER IN THE BOWL!

- Add the ingredients you need to melt to the bowl, turn the heat on medium, and watch the magic happen!

- Be careful not to get the contents of the bowl wet. (This is why you pour the water around the jar before adding the ingredients.) I like to play it safe at cover the top of the bowl with a small plate.

SCRUBS, SCRUBS, AND MORE SCRUBS

Making your own face and/or body scrub is incredibly easy. It takes less than 5 minutes to whip up a batch of scrub that will leave you feeling like you just spent a day at the spa getting pampered. You can double, triple, or quadruple the recipe and a make these scrubs for birthday gifts, holiday gifts, or "just because" gifts.

INGREDIENT NOTES

You can use salt or sugar when making a scrub. Sugar is typically gentler on the skin, especially if you have any scrapes or cuts. Salt will sting a bit when it comes in contact with broken skin.

When selecting a salt or sugar, you will want to give careful consideration to the granule size. Smaller granules (such as a finely ground sea salt or refined sugar) will be the most gentle on the skin. Unrefined gray Celtic sea salt and turbinado sugar are best for heavy exfoliation. If you have super sensitive skin, you might opt for a dark brown sugar.

When you initially mix your salt/sugar and oil, the salt/sugar might settle on the bottom. This is normal. Don't panic! You have not done anything wrong. Most scrubs will need a little stir before use.

If the scrub is a bit too oily for your tastes, add more salt/sugar. Conversely, if the scrub seems too dry, add a tad more oil. While there is a pretty standard ratio of oil to salt or sugar that I prefer to use, it can vary depending on the granule size and sometimes even the brand of salt or sugar.

TOOLS OF THE TRADE

When making a scrub, there are a few tools that are critical to its success:

- A glass bowl
- A non-wooden spoon (wood soaks up the essential oils)
- Measuring cups
- Glass jars with lids

How To Make

Unless otherwise noted, all scrubs will follow these basic directions:

1. Measure out and pour your salt or sugar into a glass bowl.
2. Slowly pour in the oil, stirring as you pour.
3. Continue to stir until the oil and salt or sugar are well blended.
4. Add the essential oils and/or spices and continue to stir.
5. Pour into your glass jars, seal, and label.

How To Use

Through experimentation, I have found that scrubs do their best work when applied to dry skin. Yes, you read that right. Apply your scrub before you turn on the shower or get into the bathtub.

I love to use a good loofah mitt or exfoliating gloves if I am going for exfoliation. Otherwise, you can apply it with your hands.

All you need is a heaping spoonful of the scrub. Place it into your palms or on your mitt/gloves and then rub the mixture all over your body in a circular motion. For tougher areas such as the knees, elbows, and soles of the feet, spend extra time scrubbing them. On places like the chest, neck, and stomach (where the skin is thinner), take a gentler approach to scrubbing. Once your entire body is scrubbed well, rinse thoroughly.

After you bathe, pat your skin dry. You probably will not need additional moisturizer but feel free to apply one of my skin moisturizing lotions for extra moisture and health benefits!

Be sure to wipe the excess oil from the shower or bathtub floor. You do not want to slip next time you bathe!

Scrub Storage

I use up my scrubs rather quickly, so I keep them in the shower. I have never had an issue with rancidity. However, I know many a scrub user who likes to play it safe, so they keep their scrubs in the refrigerator. It really is your choice. If you are not likely to use the scrub within 2-3 weeks, then I suggest storing it in the fridge.

THE SCRUBS

COCONUT LIME SCRUB

This is just a fun, refreshing scrub that is perfect for hot summer weather! It transports you to a tropical paradise.

Ingredients

- 2 cups salt or sugar
- 1 cup coconut oil, melted
- 4 tablespoons lime juice, fresh
- Zest of 1 lime

Follow basic directions adding the zest at the end and mixing well.

COCONUT OIL & HONEY FACE SCRUB

This is a simple scrub that is great for all skin types! The honey and coconut are especially nourishing, making them especially effective on dry and sensitive skin.

Ingredients

- 1 teaspoon coconut oil (melted)
- 2 tablespoons coconut milk
- 1 teaspoon honey
- 1 tablespoon brown sugar per wash

Special Directions

1. Mix coconut oil, coconut milk, and honey in a bowl.
2. Store mixture in a glass jar in a cool, dark place.
3. When ready to cleanse face, add one tablespoon of brown sugar to 1/2 tablespoon of the oil mixture.
4. Apply to skin in a circular motion for a minute or two.
5. Rinse with a warm cloth and water.

CRANBERRY SUGAR OATMEAL FACE SCRUB

The antioxidants in this scrub make it great for mature skin as well as skin that has some sun damage. You can use this daily and simply triple the batch, storing the extra in your refrigerator.

Ingredients

- 1/2 cup frozen cranberries
- 1/4 cup coconut oil
- 1/4 cup sugar
- 2 tablespoons (+ more if needed) oat powder or ground oatmeal

Special Directions

1. In a food processor, process all ingredients for 30 seconds.
2. Apply to body with gentle circular motions.
3. Makes enough for 1 shower or bath.

GREEN TEA SCRUB

The antioxidants in this scrub are quite high, making this a very thera-peutic scrub. If your skin has recently sustained any sort of sun damage, this scrub is an excellent choice. Just choose sugar and not salt if using on skin that is still slightly raw.

Ingredients

- 2 cups salt or sugar
- 1/4 cup coconut oil, melted
- 3/4 cup raw honey
- 2 tablespoons green tea
- 5 drops vanilla extract

Special Directions

1. Measure out and pour the salt or sugar into a glass bowl.
2. Slowly pour in the oil, stirring as you pour.
3. Continue to stir until the oil and salt or sugar are well blended then add in the honey.
4. Stir well to incorporate the honey.
5. Add the green tea and vanilla and continue to stir.
6. Pour into glass jars, seal, and label.

Heavy Duty Scrub

This scrub is designed to dig deep and scrub away dry, flaky skin patches. Do not use this scrub on sensitive areas like the face, and limit use to two times per week. This make an excellent scrub for callused feet!

Ingredients

- 1/2 cup salt
- 1 cup sugar
- 1/4 cup Epsom Salt
- 1/2 cup coconut oil, melted
- 1/2 cup olive oil
- 15 drops of any essential oil (EO) of your choice

Follow basic directions.

Honey Lemon Sugar Scrub

This recipe is another all-around great scrub. However, it is really beneficial to use on skin that has a lot of sunspots, freckles, and light scars from chickenpox or blemishes. It helps fade spots and even out skin tone.

Ingredients

- 1/2 cup brown sugar
- 1/2 cup salt
- 1 tablespoon lemon juice
- 1 tablespoon coconut oil (melted)
- 1 tablespoon honey

Directions

1. Follow basic directions then add lemon juice, coconut oil and honey continuing to mix well.
2. Use 1-2 times per week for amazingly smooth skin!

Lavender Rose Scrub

This scrub is excellent for mature skin as well as skin compromised by eczema or other dermatitis. It is very soothing both physically and emotionally.

Ingredients

- 1 cup salt or sugar
- 1/4 cup coconut oil, melted
- 1/4 cup almond oil
- 6 drops rosewood EO
- 4 drops lavender EO

Follow basic directions.

Mocha Spice Sugar Scrub

This is one of my favorite scrubs! It smells incredible, feels luxurious, and leaves a nice, light "tan" behind. With this scrub, you'll get the double benefit of both a nourishing scrub and a bronzer.

Ingredients

- 1 cup brown sugar
- 1/2 cup coconut oil, melted
- 1/2 cup grapeseed oil
- 1 tablespoon ground coffee
- 1 tablespoon cocoa powder
- 1 teaspoon cinnamon or 4 drops cinnamon EO
- 1/2 teaspoon nutmeg
- 1/2 teaspoon ginger

Special Directions

1. Measure out and pour the salt or sugar into a glass bowl.
2. Slowly pour in the oil, stirring as you pour.
3. Continue to stir until the oil and salt or sugar are well blended.
4. Add the ground coffee and cocoa powder and continue to stir until there are no lumps.
5. Add in the spices and stir well to incorporate.
6. Pour into glass jars, seal, and label.

Southern Peach Pie Scrub

This is another fun scrub with an amazing fragrance that brightens up your day! This scrub is made in a small batch and needs to be used within 10 days. Please store this in your refrigerator.

Ingredients

- 1/3 cup brown sugar
- 1/3 cup coconut oil, melted
- 1/4 cup almond oil
- 1 large very ripe peach, unpeeled, sliced and mashed

Follow basic directions, adding the peach in at the end and mixing well.

In addition to some of the more therapeutic scrubs, I thought it would be fin to create several "holiday themed" scrubs. These are perfect for gift-giving and are sure to elicit many "oohs" and "ahhs."

PUMPKIN PIE SCRUB

This recipe works best with the sugar blend called for but by all means, if you are a salt fan, feel free to substitute with it. This scrub smells so yummy that you will be very tempted to eat it! I have found that the light scent lingers all day and when I use it, I get compliments from strangers walking by me.

Ingredients

- 1 1/2 cups brown sugar
- 1/2 cup white sugar
- 1/2 cup coconut oil, melted
- 1/2 cup almond oil
- 1 teaspoon cinnamon or 5 drops cinnamon EO
- 1 teaspoon pumpkin pie spice
- 1/2 teaspoon nutmeg

Follow basic directions.

CANDY CANE SCRUB

This scrub is an excellent pick-me-up for those days when you are feeling fatigued. It is also wonderful to use if you have a fever or headache.

Ingredients

- 2 cups salt or sugar
- 1/2 cup coconut oil, melted
- 1/2 cup almond oil
- 10 drops peppermint EO
- A splash of beet or strawberry juice to create a red tint (optional)

Follow basic directions.

GINGERBREAD COOKIE SCRUB

I love this scrub! It smells divine and truly is a great emotional pick-me-up.

Ingredients

- 2 cups turbinado sugar
- 1/2 cup coconut oil, melted
- 1/4 cup hazelnut or almond oil
- 1 tablespoon blackstrap molasses
- 1/2 teaspoon ginger powder
- 1/4 teaspoon cinnamon or 2 drops cinnamon EO
- 1/4 teaspoon clove powder or 2 drops clove EO

Follow basic directions.

CHOCOLATE TRUFFLE LOVE SCRUB

This scrub makes a luxurious Valentine's Day scrub. I'll let you figure out how best to use it.

Ingredients

- 1 cup sugar
- 1/4 cup coconut oil, melted
- 1/4 cup almond oil
- 1/4 cup hazelnut oil
- 1/2 ounce cocoa butter
- 1/2 teaspoon cocoa powder (unsweetened)
- 1 teaspoon Vitamin E
- 1/2 teaspoon vanilla extract or 5 drops vanilla EO

Special Directions

1. Pour the sugar into a glass bowl and then mix in the oils, including the Vitamin E and vanilla. Mix well.

2. Add the cocoa powder, continuing to mix until there are no lumps.

3. Using a double boiler over medium heat, gently melt the cocoa butter, stirring constantly. Do not overheat the cocoa butter.

4. Slowly pour the cocoa butter into the scrub mixture making sure you distribute it evenly.

5. Pour into jars, let cool, then seal with a lid.

FACE AND BODY WASH

I love multi-use products, especially those that I use in the shower. It eliminates clutter and shaves a few seconds off of my personal hygiene routine.

A great face and body wash can truly make or break a shower. That squeaky clean feeling coupled with therapeutic benefits is often all it takes to start the day off right.

I have created five different face and body wash combinations, each addressing a different skin type. If you have combination skin, the face and body wash for all skin types is perfect or you can make batches of two or three of the different washes and alternate use.

The recipes below call for liquid castile or coconut soap. (Check Appendix B: Where to Purchase Quality Ingredients for brands I love). I prefer to make my own liquid coconut soap and have provided that recipe in Appendix A: Bonus Recipes).

FACE AND BODY WASH FOR ALL SKIN TYPES

Ingredients

- 1 cup liquid castile or coconut soap
- 1 tablespoon coconut oil, melted
- 2 teaspoons olive oil
- 3 drops rose EO
- 5 drops lavender EO

Directions

1. Add all ingredients to a bottle that has a lid and shake until everything is mixed well.
2. Shake before each use and apply all over body with hands, washcloth, or bath poof.

FACE AND BODY WASH FOR DRY SKIN

This face and body wash is excellent for dry or otherwise compromised skin. If you suffer from any type of dermatitis, this face and body wash will provide much needed moisture along with soothing, healing properties.

Ingredients

- 1 cup liquid castile or coconut soap
- 1/2 cup rose water
- 2 tablespoons coconut oil, melted
- 10 drops lavender EO
- 10 drops geranium EO

Directions

1. Add all ingredients to a bottle that has a lid and shake until everything is mixed well.
2. Shake before each use and apply all over body with hands, washcloth, or bath poof.

FACE AND BODY WASH FOR MATURE SKIN

Ingredients

- 1 cup liquid castile or coconut soap
- 1 tablespoon coconut oil, melted
- 2 teaspoons Vitamin E oil
- 3 drops rose EO
- 5 drops neroli EO

Directions

1. Add all ingredients to a bottle that has a lid and shake until everything is mixed well.
2. Shake before each use and apply all over body with hands, washcloth, or bath poof.

FACE AND BODY WASH FOR OILY SKIN

Ingredients

- 2 tablespoons sunflower seed, jojoba, or almond oil
- 1 tablespoon coconut oil, melted
- 2 tablespoons liquid castile or coconut soap
- 2 tablespoons aloe vera juice
- 1 tablespoon glycerin
- 2 drops lemon EO
- 2 drops sweet orange EO

Directions

1. Add all ingredients to a bottle that has a lid and shake until everything is mixed well.
2. Shake before each use and apply all over body with hands, washcloth, or bath poof.

The mixture should last for a month if stored at room temperature away from direct heat.

FACE AND BODY WASH FOR SENSITIVE SKIN

Ingredients

- 1 cup liquid castile or coconut soap
- 1/2 cup rose water
- 2 tablespoons coconut oil, melted
- 10 drops chamomile EO
- 10 drops rose EO

Directions

1. Add all ingredients to a bottle that has a lid and shake until everything is mixed well.
2. Shake before each use and apply all over body with hands, washcloth, or bath poof.

Bath Luxuries

Basic Bath Salts

This is a VERY soothing bath soak, making it great for aching muscles, menstrual cramps, sprains, strains, and pretty much anything that ails you.

Ingredients

- 3 cups Dead Sea Salt, regular sea salt, or Epsom Salt (the courser the salt, the longer it will take to dissolve in the bath)
- 1 tablespoon coconut oil, melted
- 15-20 drops of your favorite EO or EO blend

Directions

1. Place the salt mixture into a bowl.
2. Add the coconut oil and mix well with a spoon or fork.
3. Add the drops of your chosen essential oils and mix thoroughly.
4. Add the mixture to a glass jar or container that has a tight fitting lid. (Salts that are kept in a container that is not airtight will lose their aroma more quickly.)
5. Let the mixture sit for 48 hours, then mix it again to ensure that the oils are well incorporated.

To Use

Add up to one cup of salts to running bath water. Mix well to ensure that the bath salts have dispersed well in the tub, then take a relaxing bath!

BATH MELTS

Ingredients

- 2 teaspoons cocoa butter
- 4 teaspoons coconut oil
- 4 teaspoons almond oil
- 1 teaspoon jojoba oil
- 10 drops of any EO of your choice
- 1/4 teaspoon vanilla extract

Directions

1. Using the mason jar method, melt the cocoa butter and coconut oil together. Then add the almond and jojoba oils.
2. Allow to cool slightly.
3. Pour into a ceramic or glass bowl and add your choice of essential oils and vanilla. Mix well.
4. Pour the mixture into candy molds or into a shallow baking dish lined with parchment paper.
5. Place into the refrigerator for a few hours to harden. If using candy molds, pop them out and store them in a glass container or plastic bag. If using a shallow dish lined with parchment paper, cut the bath melts into squares and store them in a glass container or plastic bag.
6. Ideally, you will want to keep these bath melts in the refrigerator so they do not melt before hitting the bath water. However, if you have a place to store the melts that stays cool, they do not have to be refrigerated.

To Use

Fill your bathtub with water, then add the bath melt before getting in. It will dissolve quickly.

CHOCOLATE BATH DREAM CREAM

You will not want to get out of this bath! The rich smells of cocoa powder and cocoa butter join forces with the sweet smell of apricot and vanilla to surround you in aromatic luxury! Your skin will feel luxuriously soft and smooth after a soak in the dream cream!

Ingredients

- 1 cup cocoa powder
- 1 cup cocoa butter
- 1 cup apricot oil
- 1/2 cup coconut oil
- 1 cup of glycerin soap
- 1 teaspoon vanilla extract

Directions

1. Using the mason jar method, heat the cocoa butter until melted, then add the oils.
2. Blend with a stick blender or mixer on high.
3. While blending, drizzle in the glycerin soap and vanilla.
4. Spoon the mixture into jars and allow to cool overnight.

To Use

Add 1-2 tablespoons to your bath, under hot running water.

LAVENDER-COCONUT OIL BATH TRUFFLES

Ingredients

- 2 tablespoons white sugar
- 2 tablespoons dried lavender (or herb of choice)
- 1/2 cup coconut oil, melted
- 2 tablespoons honey
- 1/3 cup baking soda
- 3 tablespoons sea salt
- 12 drops lavender EO

Directions

1. In a clean spice or coffee grinder, combine the sugar and lavender buds.

2. In a stainless steel or glass bowl, blend the sugar-lavender mixture with the remaining ingredients. Refrigerate for one hour.

3. Using a metal spoon, scoop a generous tablespoon into your hands and mold into a ball. Place ball onto a parchment-lined baking sheet. Repeat about 12 times, or until the mixture is gone.

4. Put sheet into the refrigerator for several hours, until truffles are firm.
Store in an airtight container. (For firmer truffles, store in the fridge or a cool place.)

To Use

Place one or two of the truffles in warm bath water and enjoy.

FROTHY BATH OIL

Ingredients

- 2 eggs
- 1 cup coconut oil, melted
- 1/2 cup olive oil
- 1/2 cup almond oil
- 1 cup coconut milk
- 2 tablespoons honey
- 1/2 cup vodka
- 1 tablespoon castile or coconut soap flakes
- 3 drops EO of your choice

Directions

1. Beat together eggs, vegetable oils, and honey.
2. Add milk, vodka, soap flakes, and essential oil, still beating.
3. Pour into jars or bottles, cover, and store in the refrigerator.

To Use

Add about one tablespoon under the faucet when running the water for a warm bath.

Luxurious Bath Soak Cubes

Ingredients

- 1/3 cup cocoa butter
- 1 tablespoon coconut crème
- 1 teaspoon coconut oil
- 1 teaspoon almond oil
- 1 tablespoon honey
- 1 tablespoon powdered oatmeal
- 2 drops tangerine EO

Directions

1. Using the mason jar method, melt the cocoa butter and remove from heat.
2. Mix creamed coconut, coconut oil, almond oil, honey and oatmeal in a separate bowl and blend well.
3. Add mixture to melted cocoa butter, blend well.
4. Add tangerine essential oil (or your favorite essential oil) and blend in.
5. Pour mixture into ice cube trays and chill until firm.
6.

To Use

Toss one cube into a tub of running water and enjoy!

Soothing Bath Cookies

Ingredients

- 2 cups fine grain sea salt
- 1/2 cup baking soda
- 1/2 cup cornstarch or arrowroot powder
- 2 tablespoons coconut oil
- 2 eggs
- 6 drops EO of your choice

Directions

1. Mix ingredients until a dough forms.
2. Roll out dough and cut with small cookie cutters if desired. Otherwise, make small half dollar sized balls and flatten them slightly.
3. Bake at 350 degrees for 10 minutes.
4. Let cool. Use 1-2 cookies per bath.

ROCK THAT BODY

AFTER SUN BODY LOTION

This after-sun lotion is nourishing and quickly absorbed into parched skin. Lavender and chamomile are notoriously beneficial for any type of burn, including sunburns. They offer immediate relief and healing, and may also accelerate the healing process. Peppermint is very cooling to the skin, and therefore very beneficial for relieving sunburned skin.

Ingredients

- 1/2 cup cocoa butter
- 1/4 cup coconut oil
- 1 teaspoon almond oil
- 15 drops lavender and/or chamomile EO
- 3 drops peppermint EO

Directions

1. Place the cocoa butter, coconut oil, and almond oil in a mason jar over medium heat until butter is melted and heated for 15 minutes.
2. Pour into a cream jar and allow to cool until soft set.
3. Stir in essential oils then allow to cool completely before using.
4. Massage a small amount over body immediately after sun exposure to soothe sun parched skin.

ANTI-AGING CREAM

This lotion restores and elasticity of the skin and reduces degeneration of the skin cells.

Ingredients

- 2 tablespoons mango butter
- 2 tablespoons grated beeswax or beeswax pastilles
- 1/2 cup coconut oil
- 10 drops carrot seed oil

Directions

1. Using the mason jar method, melt the mango butter and beeswax together, stirring often.
2. Add the coconut oil, continuing to stir until everything is melted and well blended.
3. Let it cool for about 20 minutes.
4. Slowly stir in the carrot seed oil.
5. Stir until the mixture becomes a smooth paste.
6. Transfer to a glass jar with a lid and allow to harden.
7. Store in a cool dry place.
8. Use daily on face, neck, and décolletage.

BASIC SOOTHING WHIPPED BODY LOTION

Ingredients

- 1/4 cup cocoa butter
- 1 cup shea butter
- 2 tablespoons coconut oil
- 1 tablespoon jojoba oil
- 1 tablespoon almond oil
- 1/4 teaspoon Vitamin E oil (or 1 capsule)
- 1 teaspoon cornstarch or arrowroot powder (optional but it reduces the "greasy" feeling)
- Up to 20 drops of any combination of EOs (optional)

Directions

Use these cooking directions – not the mason jar method

1. Put about an inch of water in the bottom of a medium-sized pot and heat to a low simmer.

2. Place the cocoa and shea butter in a large heatproof glass measuring cup (such as Pyrex.) Place the measuring cup in the water and warm slowly over low heat until the butters are melted.

3. Cook on low heat for about 20 minutes. Do not allow to boil (or even simmer!).

4. Remove from the heat and add the remaining ingredients. Stir to combine.

5. Using an electric hand mixer, whip the butter continually for several minutes (just like you would frosting.) It will start to look like whipped cream. The more you whip it, the lighter it will become.

6. Let the mixture sit for several hours to cool and set. As it's setting, whip every couple of hours until the mixture has set to the correct texture.

7. Spoon into glass jars. To reduce air bubbles, tap the jar sharply on the counter occasionally as you're filling it. Makes about 8 ounces of whipped body lotion.

BUMP SOOTHING LOTION

Do you suffer from Keratosis Pilaris? Get rid of those bumpy red patches for good! This incredibly simple recipe will send those bumps packing.

Ingredients

- 1 cup apple cider vinegar
- 1 cup coconut oil, melted
- 2 tablespoons raw honey

Directions

1. Mix the three ingredients together and store in a glass jar.
2. Stir before using and apply to your bumpy patches daily.

CELLULITE CREAM

Ingredients

- 1/2 cup coconut oil, melted
- 1/2 cup jojoba oil
- 10 drops cypress EO
- 10 drops juniper EO
- 5 drops lavender EO

Directions

1. Mix the above oils together.
2. Massage into the affected area of the body.

Dry Skin Relief Lotion #1

Ingredients

- 3/4 cup almond oil
- 1/3 cup coconut oil
- 1 teaspoon lanolin
- 1/2 ounce grated beeswax or beeswax pastilles
- 2/3 cup rosewater
- 1/3 cup aloe vera gel
- 4 drops frankincense EO
- 4 drops helichrysum EO
- 4 drops patchouli EO
- 4 drops sandalwood EO
- 1 Vitamin E capsule

Directions

1. Using the mason jar method, melt the coconut oil, lanolin, and beeswax. Mix well and let cool.
2. In a separate bowl, mix the rosewater, aloe vera gel, and essential oils.
3. Add the contents of the vitamin E capsule to the rosewater mixture.
4. Using a handheld or stand mixer on medium-low, whip the rosewater mixture into the beeswax mixture until well blended.
5. Store in a glass jar with a tight lid.

DRY SKIN RELIEF LOTION #2

Ingredients

- 3/4 cup almond oil
- 1/3 cup coconut oil
- 1 teaspoon lanolin
- 1/2 ounce grated beeswax or beeswax pastilles
- 2/3 cup rosewater
- 1/3 cup aloe vera gel
- 2 drops rose EO
- 2 drops ylang ylang EO
- 1 vitamin E capsule

Directions

1. Using the mason jar method, melt the almond oil, coconut oil, lanolin, and beeswax. Mix well and let cool.
2. In a separate bowl, mix the rosewater, aloe vera gel, and essential oils.
3. Add the contents of the vitamin E capsule to the rosewater mixture.
4. Using a handheld or stand mixer on medium-low, whip the rosewater mixture into the beeswax mixture until well blended.
5. Store in a glass jar with a tight lid.

Lotion Bar (Customizable)

Lotion bars are a fun way to moisturize! It breaks up the monotony of applying lotions and creams. This recipe is for a basic lotion bar which you can customize with any essential oils of your choice!

Ingredients

- 1/2 cup coconut oil
- 1/2 cup shea butter or cocoa butter
- 1/2 cup grated beeswax or beeswax pastilles
- 1 teaspoon Vitamin E oil
- Up to 25 drops of your favorite EOs

Directions

1. Using the mason jar method, add all the ingredients *except the essential oils* into your jar.
2. Turn the heat on medium and bring the water around the jar to a gentle boil.
3. Stir the ingredients constantly until they are melted and there are no lumps of butter or beeswax.
4. Remove from heat, let cool for a few minutes, and stir in the essential oils.
5. Pour the mixture into molds of a shallow baking dish lined with parchment paper.
6. Allow the bars to cool completely before removing them from the molds or cutting them into squares.

MATURE SKIN OVERNIGHT LOTION

This lotion is quite heavy, which makes it a great overnight lotion. The frankincense essential oil in conjunction with the coconut oil and Vitamin E oil have been known to reduce the appearance of wrinkles and give the face a younger, plumper appearance.

Ingredients

- 2 tablespoons cocoa butter
- 1/4 cup coconut oil
- 2 tablespoons shea butter
- 2 drops frankincense EO
- 1 capsule Vitamin E oil
- 1/4 teaspoon sea salt

Directions

1. Using the mason jar method, melt the cocoa butter, shea butter, and coconut oil.
2. Stir in the sea salt until it dissolves.
3. Add frankincense and Vitamin E oil. Let cool.
4. Apply sparingly to face and leave on overnight.

MUSCLE SOOTHER

Ingredients

- 4 teaspoons shea butter
- 3 tablespoons coconut oil
- 2 tablespoons jojoba oil
- 6 drops peppermint EO
- 6 drops eucalyptus EO
- 4 drops of lavender EO
- 1 teaspoon grated beeswax or beeswax pastilles pellets

Directions

1. Using the mason jar method, melt the shea butter, coconut oil, and jojoba oil.
2. When it is liquid, add essential oils and pour into a 4oz container and let set.
3. It will be a thin ointment that will relieve tired muscles.

SCAR DIMINISHING LOTION

Ingredients

- 7 teaspoons cocoa butter
- 2 teaspoons coconut oil
- 2 teaspoons jojoba oil
- 1 teaspoon rosehip EO
- 5 drops frankincense EO
- 4 drops lavender EO

Directions

1. Using the mason jar method, melt the cocoa butter and coconut oil.
2. When it's melted, mix in the jojoba and rosehip oils.
3. As the mixture cools, mix in essential oils.
4. Let it sit overnight.
5. Use on scars twice a day, or as a basic moisturizer.

SENSITIVE SKIN OIL

Ingredients

- 2 tablespoons grapeseed oil
- 2 tablespoons coconut oil, melted
- 1 teaspoon jojoba oil
- 1 teaspoon apricot kernel oil
- 12 drops of lavender EO OR 2 drops each of jasmine and rose EOs

Directions

1. Put all the ingredients into a small glass jar with a lid and shake very well until well mixed.
2. Shake before each use.

About Face

Be sure to check out my "Rock That Body" section for more lotion recipes that work as both a face and body lotion.

Combination Skin Moisturizer

Ingredients

- 1-2 tablespoons grated beeswax or beeswax pastilles (For a lighter moisturizer, use less beeswax; for a thicker moisturizer, use more beeswax.)
- 1/4 cup coconut oil
- 1/4 cup jojoba oil
- 1 tablespoon aloe vera juice
- 1/3 cup rosewater or distilled water
- 1 teaspoon Vitamin E
- 5 drops lavender EO
- 2 drops jasmine EO
- 3 drops ylang ylang EO

Directions

1. Using the mason jar method, melt the beeswax, coconut oil, and jojoba oil into your jar.
2. Stir the ingredients constantly until they are melted and there are no lumps of beeswax.
3. Remove the jar from the pot and set aside to cool slightly.
4. While the oil and wax mixture cools, gently warm the rosewater and aloe vera juice over low heat until it is just warm to the touch.
5. Add the Vitamin E oil to the oil/wax mixture and stir well.
6. Add the rosewater and aloe vera mixture to the oil/wax and stir for about 2 minutes with a wire whisk. You want the mixture to thicken up slightly.
7. Stir in the essential oils.
8. Pour the moisturizer into a glass jar and put the lid on. For the next 3 hours, stir it 3-4 times. This will prevent the mixture from separating.

DARK CIRCLE EYE CREAM

Ingredients

- 1/4 cup peeled potato
- 1 tablespoon green tea leaves
- 1 teaspoon coconut oil, melted

Directions

1. Process until smooth in a food processor or blender.
2. Apply under eyes at night after cleansing.
3. Leave on all night.
4. Refrigerate unused portion and use within 14 days.

GREEN GODDESS FACE MASK

Ingredients

- 1 cup sliced fresh carrot root
- 2 cups fresh spinach leaves
- 1/2 cup sliced mushrooms
- 2 cups fresh, sliced zucchini squash
- 1/2 cup vegetable water (left over from steaming veggies)
- 2 tablespoons coconut oil, melted
- 1/2 cup French green clay

Directions

1. Combine all the vegetables and steam until soft and tender.
2. Let vegetables cool completely and save 1/2 cup of their cooking water.
3. Put the water and veggies in blender or food processor and process until smooth, pale green and creamy. Using a whisk or fork, stir in the clay and coconut oil.
4. When finished, spread a thick layer of the creamy mask all over your face using a small paintbrush.
5. Let the mask sit on your skin for 10-15 minutes. Rinse off mask with warm water.
6. Store in a glass jar in the refrigerator and use within 14 days. (Makes enough for 4 treatments.)

HYDRATING FACE SPRAY

This is the best pick-me-up for a down-and-out face. Use this on tired, dry, chapped skin or on skin that suddenly developed an oil slick. It calms, soothes, and fortifies!

Ingredients

- 1 cup distilled water or rose water
- 10 drops of any EO(s) of your choosing
- 1/2 teaspoon glycerin
- 1/2 teaspoon coconut oil, melted
- If you have oily, blemish-prone skin, try adding a teaspoon of natural witch hazel

Directions

1. Pour all the ingredients into a jar and shake vigorously until well blended. Once mixed, pour the concoction into a spray bottle.
2. Spray as often as needed to refresh and hydrate the face.

MAKEUP REMOVER

Ingredients

- 1 tablespoon castor oil
- 1 tablespoon coconut oil, melted
- 2 teaspoons olive oil
- 1 drop grapefruit EO

Directions

1. Blend the oils together and place in a glass jar.
2. Apply to your face, remove with a warm, damp cloth, and rinse.
3. Can be used to remove eye makeup too!

OILY SKIN COMBAT LOTION

Ingredients

- 1/4 cup coconut oil
- 1/4 cup almond, grapeseed, or olive oil
- 1 teaspoon shea butter
- 1/2 teaspoon jojoba oil
- 2 tablespoons grated beeswax or beeswax pastilles
- 1/2 teaspoon honey
- 1/4 cup distilled water mixed with 1/4 teaspoon of baking soda
- 10 drop palmarosa EO
- 3 drops tea tree EO
- 5 drops lemongrass EO

Directions

1. Using the mason jar method, melt the oils (*except the essential oils*) and beeswax. Transfer to a large glass bowl.

2. In a separate small pot, bring the water and baking soda to a gentle boil and remove from heat.

3. Slowly pour the water mixture into the melted oil and beeswax mixture.

4. Using a wire whisk or hand blender, beat the mixture until slightly cool.

5. Add the essential oils and continue beating until a creamy texture is formed to your liking.

6. If the mixture is not thick enough, simply melt and add a little more beeswax.

7. Transfer to glass jars for storage.

8. Use twice daily on oily skin to help balance the sebum glands on your face.

REJUVENATING FACE CLEANSER

Ingredients

- 6 tablespoons flaxseed oil
- 6 tablespoons olive oil
- 3/4 cup coconut oil, melted
- 30 drops EOs of your choice

Directions

1. Add flaxseed oil, coconut oil, and olive oils to a bottle or jar.
2. Add essential oils.
3. Gently shake to blend before each use.
4. Apply a small amount to face and massage to cleanse. Rinse with warm water and a wash cloth.

LOVE THOSE LOCKS

One of the areas where many people are hesitant to make their own personal care products is in the shampoo and conditioner realm. We are so used to commercial products that create thick, rich lathers, that making the switch to shampoos that are less sudsy and conditioners that are more oily is a rather big adjustment. However, your hair will thank you for allowing it to be free from all those harsh chemicals that strip all the wonderful hair oils out while adding back in synthetic moisture.

SHAMPOOS

Dry Hair Shampoo

Ingredients

- 2 cups water
- 1 cup coconut milk
- 1/4 cup coconut oil
- 3/4 cup grated castile or coconut soap
- 12 drops rose, chamomile, red clover, or comfrey EO

Directions

This recipe works best using the double boiler method

1. In a double boiler add the water, coconut milk, coconut oil, and castile soap.
2. Cook over low heat until the ingredients have melted.
3. Blend in the essential oils.
4. Pour into jars and let cool.

Oily Hair Shampoo

Ingredients

- 3 cups water
- 1/4 cup coconut oil
- 3/4 cup grated castile or coconut soap
- 12 drops yarrow, lemon balm, or thyme EO

Directions

This recipe works best using the double boiler method

1. In a double boiler add the water, coconut oil, and castile soap.
2. Cook over low heat until the ingredients have melted.
3. Blend in the essential oils.
4. Pour into jars and let cool.

Shampoo for All Hair Types

Ingredients

- 3 cups water
- 1/4 cup coconut oil
- 3/4 cup grated castile or coconut soap
- 12 drops parsley, linden (lime flower), or rosemary EO

Directions

This recipe works best using the double boiler method

1. In a double boiler add the water, coconut oil, and castile soap.
2. Cook over low heat until the ingredients have melted.
3. Blend in the essential oils.
4. Pour into jars and let cool.

Shampoo for Blondes

Ingredients

- 3 cups water
- 1/4 cup coconut oil
- 3/4 cup grated castile or coconut soap
- 12 drops chamomile or calendula EO

Directions

This recipe works best using the double boiler method

1. In a double boiler add the water, coconut oil, and castile soap.
2. Cook over low heat until the ingredients have melted.
3. Blend in the essential oils.
4. Pour into jars and let cool.

Shampoo for Brunettes

Ingredients

- 3 cups water
- 1/4 cup coconut oil
- 3/4 cup grated castile or coconut soap
- 12 drops rosemary or sage EO

Directions

This recipe works best using the double boiler method

1. In a double boiler add the water, coconut oil, and castile soap.
2. Cook over low heat until the ingredients have melted.
3. Blend in the essential oils.
4. Pour into jars and let cool.

Deep Hair Conditioner

Ingredients

- 2 tablespoons coconut oil, melted
- 2 drops Roman chamomile EO
- 2 drops lavender EO
- 2 drops sandalwood EO
- 1 drop jasmine EO

Directions

1. Before showering, combine all of the ingredients in a glass measuring cup. Mix thoroughly.
2. Rub mixture through hair and leave on for 15 minutes.
3. Shampoo and condition as usual.

Hair Butter

Ingredients

- 2 tablespoons shea butter
- 2 tablespoons mango butter
- 2 tablespoons coconut oil
- 1 teaspoon lanolin
- 1 teaspoon almond oil
- 1 teaspoon jojoba oil
- 1 teaspoon avocado oil
- 10 drops ylang-ylang EO
- 1/8 teaspoon vanilla extract

Directions

1. Using the mason jar method, melt the butters, the lanolin, and the oils (*except the essential oils*).
2. Pour in container, add the essential oils and vanilla extract and let cool.
3. You can apply this before showering and leave on for 15 minutes. Shampoo and condition as usual.
4. Alternatively, you can use this as a conditioner after shampooing.
5. Makes about 4 one-ounce treatments.

Hair Oil Treatment

Ingredients

- 1 cup coconut oil
- 1 cup sunflower seed oil
- 1/4 cup hemp seed oil
- 2 tablespoons avocado oil
- 2 tablespoons jojoba oil
- 2 tablespoons Vitamin E oil
- 2 tablespoons cocoa butter
- 2 tablespoons avocado butter
- 2 tablespoons mango butter

Directions

1. Using the mason jar method, melt all of the ingredients.
2. Pour into a jar.
3. When ready to use, heat gently for about 10 minutes in a bowl of boiling water until liquid and warm, but not hot.
4. Apply liberally to hair and scalp, let soak for 15-20 minutes, then shampoo out.
5. A second shampooing may be required.
6. Apply treatment once a week.

Scalp Treatment Oil

Ingredients

- 3 tablespoons coconut oil, melted
- 4 teaspoons neem oil
- 1 teaspoon hemp seed oil
- 1 teaspoon borage oil
- 2-3 drops palmarosa EO
- 2-3 drops lavender EO
- 2-3 drops bergamot EO
- 2-3 drops carrot seed EO
- 2-3 drops rosemary EO
- 10 drops bay leaf EO

Directions

1. Blend and bottle the oils.
2. Shake gently and put a few drops on fingertips to massage into freshly shampooed scalp where there is scaling and flaking.
3. Protect scalp from sunlight, as bergamot can be phototoxic.

Kiss Me

Lip Balm Making 101

Here is the simple method of making lip balm:

1. Coarsely chop or grate beeswax if not using pastilles, and place in a mason jar along with the butters and carrier oils. Gently melt the ingredients together over simmering water.

2. Once the wax mixture has melted, remove the mason jar from the pot, cool for one minute, and add the essential oils. The essential oils will begin to dissipate when heated, so add more as needed. When you are happy with the scent and all ingredients are well combined, immediately pour the warm mixture into lip balm containers – either tubes or tins.

3. If the mixture cools too rapidly when pouring, simply reheat the mixture in the mason jar. Allow the balm to cool completely (usually overnight) before placing the caps on your lip balm containers.

Basic Lip Balm

Ingredients

- 2 teaspoons coconut oil
- 1 teaspoon grated beeswax or beeswax pastilles
- 1 Vitamin E capsule
- 2-3 drops flavor oil

Chocolate Peppermint Lip Balm

Ingredients

- 2 tablespoons grated beeswax or beeswax pastilles
- 1/4 cup coconut oil
- 2-3 drops carrot seed EO
- 2 tablespoons any butter of your choice (cocoa/shea/mango or a mix)
- 1/4 teaspoon honey
- 3 - 5 drops peppermint EO

COCONUT LEMON LIP BALM

Ingredients

- 1 tablespoon coconut oil
- 2 tablespoons sunflower oil
- 4 teaspoons grated beeswax or beeswax pastilles
- 10 drops lemon EO

HEALING HERBAL LIP BALM (UNSCENTED)

Ingredients

- 1 tablespoon shea butter
- 2 tablespoons calendula infused olive oil (simply place the herbs in the olive oil for two hours then strain the herbs out)
- 1 tablespoon jojoba oil
- 4 teaspoons grated beeswax or beeswax pastilles
- 5 drops Vitamin E oil

COLD SORE BALM

This cold sore balm is very effective and offers immediate relief. The peppermint essential oil is very soothing, and the coconut oil and tea tree oil get to the root of the virus, attacking it quickly.

Ingredients

- 4 tablespoons grated beeswax or beeswax pastilles
- 3 tablespoons coconut oil
- 1 tablespoon almond oil
- 5 drops tea tree EO
- 2 drops Vitamin E oil
- 2 drops peppermint EO

Directions

1. Using the mason jar method, melt the beeswax and coconut oil.
2. Remove from heat, allow to cool slightly, add the sweet almond oil, vitamin E oil, and essential oils.
3. Pour into container or jar.

ANYTHING GOES

INSECT REPELLENT LOTION

Ingredients

- 1 cup coconut oil, melted
- 2 tablespoons olive oil
- 20 drops EOs. The best insect repelling essential oils are patchouli, citronella, cedarwood, eucalyptus, lavender, and peppermint.

Directions

1. Mix all of the ingredients together and store in a jar.
2. Apply liberally all over body.

HERBAL STICK DEODORANT

Ingredients

- 2 tablespoons grated beeswax or beeswax pastilles
- 2 tablespoons cocoa butter
- 2 tablespoons coconut oil
- 2 tablespoons castor oil
- 1 teaspoon grapefruit seed extract
- 1 teaspoon tea tree EO
- 2 teaspoons lavender or orange EO
- 1 teaspoon rosemary EO
- 8 drops myrrh EO (optional)

Directions

1. Using the mason jar method, melt the oils and the beeswax.
2. Remove from heat and add the essential oils and stir.
3. Pour into a new or used deodorant container and allow to solidify.

LOVE POTION

Ingredients

- 1 tablespoon coconut oil
- 1-1/2 teaspoons honey
- 1/8 teaspoon vanilla extract

Directions

1. Using the mason jar method, add all of the ingredients, stirring until melted and combined.
2. Pour in a small container immediately, before it cools.
3. What you do with it from there is none of my concern. (It is edible).

MINT (OR FLAVOR OF CHOICE) TOOTHPASTE

Ingredients

- 2 teaspoons baking soda
- 4 teaspoons arrowroot powder
- 1/4 teaspoon sea salt
- 4 teaspoons coconut oil, melted
- 10 drops of peppermint or other EO

Directions

1. Mix ingredients well and store in a glass jar.
2. Apply toothpaste onto toothbrush and brush teeth as normal. Toothpaste can be gently stirred before using is needed.

PMS Oil Blend

Ingredients

- 1/2 cup coconut oil, melted
- 10 drops geranium EO
- 15 drops lavender EO
- 5 drops German chamomile EO
- 3 drops cypress EO

Directions

1. Mix oils together and store in a bottle or jar.
2. Apply to abdomen as needed to relieve cramps.

THERAPEUTIC MASSAGE CANDLE

This is a recipe for pure luxury! Not only do you get to enjoy safe-burning candlelight, but your body will reap the benefits. You will notice that I do not give exact measurements in the ingredient list. This is because the measurements will vary on the size of your jar. If your percentages are a wee bit off, don't worry! The candle will still turn out.

Ingredients

- 60% cocoa butter
- 30% coconut oil
- 10% sweet almond oil
- 15-20 drops of your favorite EOs (lavender, geranium, sandalwood, sweet orange, and frankincense work well)
- 1 glass jar to hold the candle
- 1 candle wick

Directions

1. On very low heat melt the cocoa butter and coconut oil in a saucepan. Do not let it boil or get too hot! Use low heat at all times.

2. Once the cocoa butter and coconut oil have melted, add the almond oil and stir in well. Let cool for 3 minutes.

3. Put 6-8 drops of essential oil at the bottom of the jar.

4. Place the candle wick in the center of the jar. While holding the wick, pour in the warm oil mix.

5. If your home is cool in temperature you can leave to set naturally. If you are keeping your home warm, find the coolest spot in the house and let the candle set.

When it is set and you are ready to use, light the candle and let the oils melt a little. Blow the candle out and pour warm oil into your hands and massage over the body. Re-light the candle when you are ready for your next massage. You can also keep it burning like a regular candle but it will melt quickly.

Wart Be-Gone

Ingredients

- 1/8 cup coconut oil, melted
- 3 drops lemon EO
- 5 drops tea tree EO
- 2 drops thyme EO

Directions

1. Mix the oils together and apply four times daily to the affected area.

2. Do not wash area for at least 30 minutes after application.

APPENDIX A: BONUS RECIPES

LIQUID COCONUT SOAP

Ingredients

- 1 - 8 ounce bar of coconut soap
- 2 tablespoons Liquid Glycerin (found in the bandge section at any drugstore or grocery store)
- 1 gallon distilled water

Directions

1. Grate the entire bar of soap. Alternatively, you can grind it up in the blender.

2. Fill a pot with one gallon of distilled water and add the soap. (Any water will work however, distilled water helps the liquid soap keep a longer shelf life).

3. Add the liquid glycerin, turn the heat to medium, and stir until the soap dissolves. This can take some time. You need to make sure that the soap is completely dissolved.

4. Remove the pot from the heat and let it stand for 12 hours.

5. After 12 hours, the soap should be a thicker consistency. Take an egg beater and gently whip it for 2 minutes.

6. Pour into containers to use in other recipes. You can also use this alone as hand soap.

APPENDIX B: WHERE TO PURCHASE INGREDIENTS

Most local health food stores will carry the ingredients listed in this eBook. If you are anything like me, you prefer to make cost saving purchases online whenever possible. More importantly, you want to source the highest quality ingredients from the most ethical, sustainable companies possible.

Below I have provided a short list of those companies with which I do business. I have vetted each company carefully and can assure you that you are not only getting the highest quality product possible but that you are also getting it for a fair price.

For links to all of the products and companies listed here, please visit http://www.hybridrastamama.com/ingredient-and-product-links.

COCONUT OIL

Tropical Traditions

This was the first coconut oil I ever tried and I knew immediately that it was an incredible oil. Tropical Traditions offers 3 different kinds of coconut oil (Gold Label Coconut Oil, Green Label Coconut Oil, and Expeller Pressed Coconut Oil). The Expeller Pressed is great to use in salves if you do not want the coconut scent infused with the herbs and essential oils you are using. All of these oils come in gallon and five gallon buckets which makes them very cost effective.

Barlean's

This is another fabulous coconut oil and I have found that I really enjoy using it when making salves that will be used on or around my face. Even though it retains the coconut oil smell, it is not overpowering.

OLIVE OIL

Tropical Traditions - This company is more than just a coconut oil manufacturer. They sell Extra Virgin Olive Oil as well. It comes in a 3 liter can and works perfectly in my salve recipes.

HERBS

Mountain Rose Herbs - This is my one stop shop for organic dried herbs. Their prices cannot be beat and they are a company whose values I can stand behind.

HONEY

If you are going to be making a lot of personal care products requiring honey, I suggest you order raw honey in bulk. The best quality raw honey for the most affordable price can be found at Tropical Traditions in a 15 pound pail.

ESSENTIAL OILS

This is a loaded topic as not every essential oil is worthy of being used in a therapeutic sense. In the case of essential oils, cheaper is not better. I have yet to find an inexpensive essential oil that is a really high quality oil in terms of distillation method, the location in which the herb was grown, and the farming practices used.

While I personally use several different brands with success, I honestly do not feel qualified to recommend an essential oil as the one that is the highest quality. Please do your own research and decide which you feel comfortable using in your salve making.

OTHER INGREDIENTS

I purchase the following ingredients from Mountain Rose Herbs:

- Beeswax, Carnauba Wax, and Soy Wax
- Castile Soap
- Lanolin
- Liquid Glycerine

I purchase the following ingredients from the Green Polka Dot Box:

- Arrowroot Powder
- Cornstarch
- Green Tea

I purchase the following ingredients from **Tropical Traditions**:

- Coconut Soap
- Apple Cider Vinegar

APPENDIX C: RESEARCH AND SOURCES

PRINT BOOKS

Virgin Coconut Oil by Brian and Marianita Shilhavy

Eat Fat Lose Fat: The Healthy Alternative to Trans Fats by Mary Enig, PhD, and Sally Fallon

The Coconut Oil Miracle Revised and Coconut Cures both by Bruce Fife.

WEBSITES

http://www.ewg.org/skindeep/

Pubmed.gov (specific articles/studies):

- http://www.ncbi.nlm.nih.gov/pubmed/11413497
- http://www.ncbi.nlm.nih.gov/pubmed/20523108
- http://www.ncbi.nlm.nih.gov/pubmed/17966176
- http://www.ncbi.nlm.nih.gov/pubmed/20523108
- http://www.ncbi.nlm.nih.gov/pubmed/19115123

JOURNAL ARTICLES

D O Ogbolu, A A Oni, O A Daini, A P Oloko. In vitro antimicrobial properties of coconut oil on Candida species in Ibadan, Nigeria. *J Med Food*. 2007 Jun;10(2):384-7. PMID: 17651080

Graciela E Hurtado de Catalfo, María J T de Alaniz, Carlos A Marra. Dietary lipids modify redox homeostasis and steroidogenic status in rat testis. *Phytother Res*. 2010 Feb;24(2):163-8. PMID: 18549927

Ian F Burgess, Elizabeth R Brunton, Nazma A Burgess . Clinical trial showing superiority of a coconut and anise spray over permethrin 0.43% lotion for head louse infestation, ISRCTN96469780. *Eur J Pediatr*. 2010 Jan ;169(1):55-62. Epub 2009 Apr 3. PMID: 19343362

K G Nevin, T Rajamohan . Effect of topical application of virgin coconut oil on skin components and antioxidant status during dermal wound healing in young rats. *Skin Pharmacol Physiol*. 2010 ;23(6):290-7. Epub 2010 Jun 3. PMID: 20523108

Lauren E Conlon, Ryan D King, Nancy E Moran, John W Erdman. Coconut Oil Enhances Tomato Carotenoid Tissue Accumulation Compared to Safflower Oil in the Mongolian Gerbil (Meriones unguiculatus). *J Agric Food Chem*. 2012 Aug 7. Epub 2012 Aug 7. PMID: 22866697

María de Lourdes Arruzazabala, Vivian Molina, Rosa Más, Daisy Carbajal, David Marrero, Víctor González, Eduardo Rodríguez. Effects of coconut oil on testosterone-induced prostatic hyperplasia in Sprague-Dawley rats. *J Pharm Pharmacol*. 2007 Jul;59(7):995-9. PMID: 17637195

Mark A Reger, Samuel T Henderson, Cathy Hale, Brenna Cholerton, Laura D Baker, G S Watson, Karen Hyde, Darla Chapman, Suzanne Craft . Effects of beta-hydroxybutyrate on cognition in memory-impaired adults. *Neurobiol Aging*. 2004 Mar;25(3):311-4. PMID: 15123336

Mouna Abdelrahman Abujazia, Norliza Muhammad, Ahmad Nazrun Shuid, Ima Nirwana Soelaiman. The Effects of Virgin Coconut Oil on Bone Oxidative Status in Ovariectomised Rat. *Evid Based Complement Alternat Med*. 2012 ;2012:525079. Epub 2012 Aug 15. PMID: 22927879

Pallavi Srivastava, S Durgaprasad. Burn wound healing property of Cocos nucifera: An appraisal. *Indian J Pharmacol*. 2008 Aug;40(4):144-6. PMID: 20040946

R O Nneli, O A Woyike. Antiulcerogenic effects of coconut (Cocos nucifera) extract in rats. *Phytother Res*. 2008 Jul;22(7):970-2. PMID: 18521965

S Intahphuak, P Khonsung, A Panthong. Anti-inflammatory, analgesic, and antipyretic activities of virgin coconut oil. *Pharm Biol*. 2010 Feb;48(2):151-7. PMID: 20645831

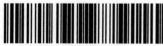

Made in the USA
San Bernardino, CA
07 October 2017